Vegan, Vegetarian, Keto, Atkins, Low-Fat, Zone, Dukan, Raw Food, Juice, Mediterranean, Military, and DASH Diets

Knowing Which Diets Are Fast and Good for Your Body to Create Long-Lasting Results

Lee Rayford

contained within this document, including, but not limited to, errors, omissions, or inaccuracies.

Table of Contents

INTRODUCTION 1

CHAPTER 1: VEGAN DIET 5

WHAT IS IT? 5

WHO CAN BENEFIT? 6

    Pros 7

    Cons 8

    Duration 9

SHOPPING LIST 10

MEAL PLAN 12

CHAPTER 2: VEGETARIAN DIET 15

WHAT IS IT? 15

WHO CAN BENEFIT? 16

    Pros 16

    Cons 17

    Duration 18

SHOPPING LIST 19

MEAL PLAN 21

CHAPTER 3: KETOGENIC DIET 25

WHAT IS IT? 25

WHO CAN BENEFIT? 27

    Pros 28

    Cons 28

    Duration 30

SHOPPING LIST 30

MEAL PLANS 32

CHAPTER 4: ATKINS DIET 39

WHAT IS IT? 39

WHO CAN BENEFIT? 41

    Pros 41

    Cons 42

    Duration 43

SHOPPING LIST 43

    Introduction Shopping List 43

Remaining Phases Shopping List 45

MEAL PLANS 46

Introduction Diet (Phase One) 46

Remainder of Diet 49

CHAPTER 5: LOW-FAT DIET **55**

WHAT IS IT? 55

WHO CAN BENEFIT? 57

Pros 57

Cons 58

Duration 59

SHOPPING LIST 60

MEAL PLAN 61

CHAPTER 6: ZONE DIET **65**

WHAT IS IT? 65

WHO CAN BENEFIT? 68

Pros 68

Cons 69

Duration 70

SHOPPING LIST 70

MEAL PLANS 72

CHAPTER 7: DUKAN DIET **83**

WHAT IS IT? 83

WHO CAN BENEFIT? 86

Pros 86

Cons 87

Duration 88

SHOPPING LIST 88

MEAL PLAN 91

CHAPTER 8: RAW FOOD DIET **97**

WHAT IS IT? 97

WHO CAN BENEFIT? 98

Pros 99

Cons 99

Duration 101

SHOPPING LIST 101

MEAL PLAN 103

CHAPTER 9: JUICE DIET **107**

WHAT IS IT? 107

WHO CAN BENEFIT? 110

Pros 110

Cons 110

Duration 111

SHOPPING LIST 113

MEAL PLANS 114

CHAPTER 10: MEDITERRANEAN DIET **119**

WHAT IS IT? 119

WHO CAN BENEFIT? 121

Pros 122

Cons 122

Duration 123

SHOPPING LIST 124

MEAL PLAN 126

CHAPTER 11: MILITARY DIET **131**

WHAT IS IT? 131

WHO CAN BENEFIT? 132

Pros 132

Cons 133

Duration 133

SHOPPING LIST 134

MEAL PLANS 137

CHAPTER 12: DASH DIET **145**

WHAT IS IT? 145

WHO CAN BENEFIT? 149

Pros 149

Cons 150

Duration 151

SHOPPING LIST 151

MEAL PLAN 153

CONCLUSION **159**

REFERENCES **163**

IMAGE REFERENCES **193**

Introduction

We have all heard the saying, "New year, new me." There are always the promises of becoming healthy when the new year rolls around, especially after gorging on delicious Christmas and New Year's treats. No one is blaming you; we have all been there. However, when the parties are all drying up and we are getting ready to get back to work, some of us may notice that our favorite dress is fitting just a little tighter, or maybe the belt needs to be taken back a notch. So, you overdid it over the holiday season, no big deal. Nothing a quick visit to the gym or a diet can't fix. Don't let that statement fool you. It isn't that easy. According to the Boston Medical Center (n.d.), approximately 45 million Americans will go on a diet every single year and can spend upward of $33 billion on products that "guarantee" weight loss. Yet, almost two-thirds of the American population is either obese or overweight. Obesity is not something that goes away by simply ignoring it. It needs to be treated and is even considered a chronic disease by medical professionals. Unless something is done about this condition, it becomes a lifelong struggle with not only extra pounds but also diseases such as high cholesterol, blood pressure, diabetes, and a variety of heart and other diseases. It is not that one can die from obesity but rather from the side effects of it.

Obesity can be managed in several ways. The most common are those of diet and exercise programs. Then, there are medical interventions such as weight-loss medications and bariatric surgery, which are any surgeries that aid in weight loss, such as gastric bypass. Some people even benefit from behavioral support groups where they come together with other like-minded people where they can focus on things such as nutrition, cooking healthy meals, as well as keeping a food diary to help find out why they eat the way that they do. This doesn't always need to be done in a group setting and can be handled by one's self if your willpower is strong enough.

Obesity can be controlled when one puts their mind to it, but you have to be willing to do the work that comes with it. It took years to pack on the extra pounds, and thus, it will take more than an overnight diet to fix it. There are many diets available today. Some are easy to stick to and some significantly more difficult. The most commonly used one by most Americans is the *Dietary Guidelines for Americans*. This guideline is ever-changing and a new version is released every five years (Health.gov, n.d.). The latest edition of this diet now provides information about a healthy diet for all life stages of people as well as for pregnant or breastfeeding women.

If one takes the time to read through the 164-page document titled *Dietary Guidelines for Americans, 2020-2025*, you will see that the diets are all tailored differently depending on age. There is not one diet that suits a person from birth to death. This is, according to Health.gov, that nutrition is not something that suits everyone all the time and that it needs to change depending on the situation. The guidelines are just that, guidelines, which allow people to make educated decisions about their food. It is for this reason that there are so many different diets available to us. There are hundreds of diets ranging from low-fat, low-sodium, high-fat, low-carb, etc. that people make use of every year to manage all sorts of problems they may have, not just obesity.

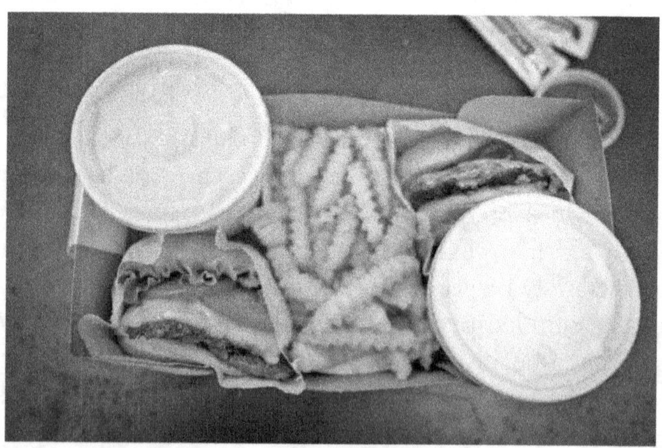

Is the convenience of junk food worth the health cost?

With that said, how do you know which diet will help you with your weight problems? First and foremost, it is vital that you talk to your physician about any changes you want to make to your diet or exercise regimen before taking the plunge. Some diets available to people may interact badly with certain medicines, body conditions, or simply may not suit you. After that, you can start by doing your research, which you have by picking up a copy of this book! Not only are 12 of the most popular diets being discussed, but all the pros and cons will be made available to allow you to make the correct decision about your health. It is suggested that you read this book from cover to cover before deciding on a diet, as each will contain a shopping list as well as a meal plan for a week, with some exceptions—certain diets shouldn't be followed longer than a few days.

Some diets are more than just that, they are lifestyles where you will need to change more than just your diet to make use of them. Then, there are others to help you make a small change to your life before reverting to a standard diet. The main message in these diets is that you will need to make some sacrifices when it comes to some of your favorite foods. So, if you have a sugar addiction, now is a good time to get rid of some of those empty-calorie treats such as sodas to make way for healthier options. All of these diets can be coupled with exercise if you so wish, though with some it may be more difficult to reach certain peaks in your training.

The important thing to remember is that your body is not a prison but rather a temple. If you want it looking good, then put a little planning into it and give it the fuel that it deserves. No one deserves to be judged for the way they look if they are working on themselves a little every day. So, take the time to educate yourself about the diets within the book and see which would suit the kind of life you lead. Little changes here and there may be all you need, or you may need a complete lifestyle change to achieve what you want.

I am Lee Rayford, and I am someone who takes pride in being an expert in wellness, health, and fitness. I want to help people incorporate wellness as a lifestyle and not a punishment. The looks people give you as you walk past is punishment enough. We are going to change those looks of judgment into looks of awe as you work on yourself to give yourself the better life you deserve. So, join me in this journey to decide which diet or lifestyle best suits what you need from it to gain maximum happiness and health.

You can either make use of the diets listed in the book as a complete lifestyle change or you can make use of it to just achieve that smaller size so your favorite clothing item fits you perfectly once again. Remember, you are not in this alone—there are at least 45 million other Americans who will be starting their dietary change journey with you. Don't be afraid to join local groups or forums if you need a little extra help to stick to the changes which may not be so easy to do. Everything is easier when you have the support, and this book is the first step. Let's get started on making a better you so that you can have a better life.

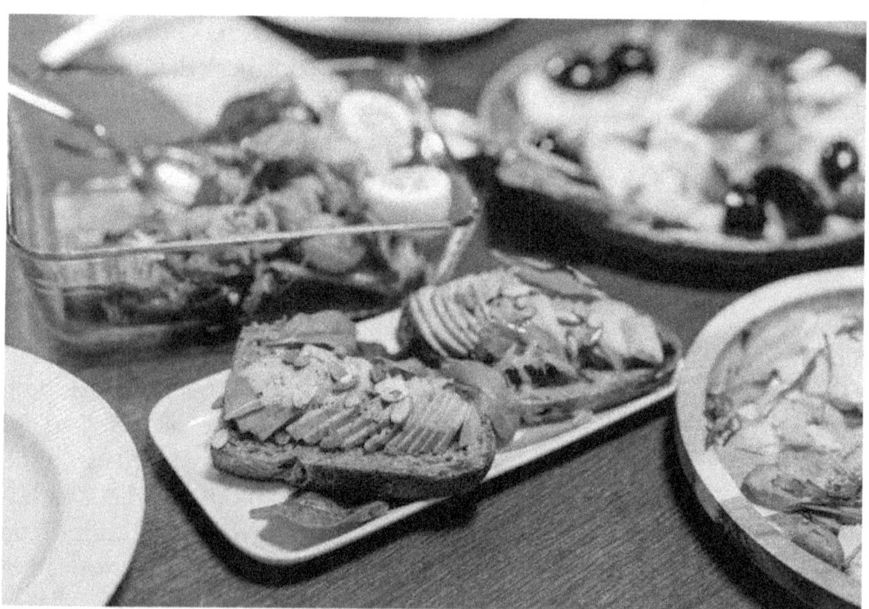

Chapter 1:

Vegan Diet

What Is It?

Let's kick off the diets with likely one of the most restrictive of the diets that one can make a change to. Veganism is a way of life where a person makes no use of animal products at all, whether the animal has been killed for the product (meat) or not (wool). This diet, and lifestyle, are becoming increasingly more popular as people are switching to it for health, ethical, and even environmental reasons (Petre, 2016). The lifestyle doesn't change but there are several vegan diets that one may utilize:

- The starch solution: High-carb diet where the focus of the diet is on cooked grains and potatoes instead of on fruit.

- Whole foods diet: Whole plant foods, seeds, fruits, vegetables, etc., and minimally processed foods.

- 80/10/10 diet: More fresh fruit and vegetables while limiting high-fat plants such as nuts and avocado.

- Raw-food diet: Whole plant foods that are consumed raw or cooked below temperatures of 118 °F.

- Plant-based/Just vegan: No strict guidelines other than not eating any animal products.

These are just a fraction of some of the diets that are available to one who wants to make use of the vegan diet. There are about 15 diets in total one may use (Alena, 2017). Others you may have heard of are the nutritarian diet, junk and convenience food diet, detox diet, SOS—sugar, oil, and salt—free plant-based diet, Raw Till Four diet, whole starch low-fat diet, high-carb low-fat diet, Esselstyn heart healthy diet, low-carb diet—can be used with ketogenic and Atkins diet—and the Engine 2 Diet. So you are quite spoiled for choice when it comes to which of the vegan diets you would like to follow.

Some of the diets are considered healthier than others, but your choice will come down to what it is you want to achieve from the diet. If you simply wish to give up on using animal-based products, then following the classic plant-based diet is the best. However, if you want to concentrate on certain macronutrients—fat, protein, and carbohydrates—then you can make use of the diets that favor one over the other.

Who Can Benefit?

Anyone and everyone who no longer wants to make use of animal-based products can benefit from the vegan diet. This becomes not only a diet but also a lifestyle change, as you will need to be more conscious about products that have been tested on animals or may have come from an animal source. It is vital for someone on a vegan diet to become acquainted with items—not just food—that could contain animal products. Marshmallows are a great example. They contain gelatin which is made from boiling animal products such as skin, tendons, bones, and ligaments. Unless the packet says vegan-friendly, always read the labels and educate yourself on terms used for animal products.

Pros

The advantages of switching to a vegan diet are numerous, despite the restrictiveness. The first and foremost, and the reason you may be reading this book, is the ability to lose weight on this diet. Even when one eats until they are full, those on a vegan diet still manage to lose weight, and it is believed that this is due to the high volumes of fiber in the diet that gives the feeling for feeling fuller for longer (Petre, 2016).

This fiber is very important as it also manages to control blood sugar (glucose) by allowing the sugar from the diet to be released slowly over time. So, even if you are someone making use of the whole foods diet, which contains a lot of fruit, the fructose will be used slowly by the body instead of giving you that instant sugar rush followed by the crash thereafter. With a lower amount of glucose in your blood, you will stand a lower chance of developing type 2 diabetes.

Animal products contain cholesterol. As you are eating less of these food items, you will find that your cholesterol will be lower than those that continue to eat animal-sourced foods. Even your blood pressure will start to improve as you get used to eating on this diet. Avoiding animal-based fats will also contribute to a healthier heart and prevent later heart diseases. Choosing plant-based proteins over animal-based proteins may also be gentler on the kidneys, as waste products of proteins are flushed through them.

Even the symptoms of arthritis are lower while there is a lower chance of catching certain types of cancers, such as colon cancer, as long as you are avoiding overly processed foods (Madigan & Karhu, 2018). There have even been some studies to show that a vegan diet can aid in slowing down the onset of Alzheimer's disease. Something else that has been noticed is that people who adopt the vegan lifestyle tend to be somewhat healthier, as they tend to quit smoking, make healthier choices when it comes to their meals, and even start exercising more (Brown, 2020).

Cons

Like everything in life, there is good as well as bad, and this is true for all diets with no exception. As with all restrictive diets, there are always some nutrients that will be lacking. With veganism, what is lacking are vitamin B12, folate, omega fatty acids, and calcium (Brown, 2020). Each of these is essential to the human body.

Many vegans lack calcium in their diets because of not balancing their diets with vegetables that contain this mineral. Because of this, vegans are more prone to lower bone density and bone breaks than any other people on other diets. It is believed that this is also caused by the lack of vitamin B12. This vitamin is crucial as it helps to prevent nerve damage. It has been noted that vegan diets, although healthy for the heart, may lead to higher risks of strokes and even hemorrhagic strokes—though to a lesser degree—because of not having this vitamin. Babies which are placed on a vegan diet—for whatever reason—will fail to thrive unless the vitamin is present. Symptoms of a lack of B12 include fatigue, feeling weak, constipation, as well as a lack of appetite (Iyer, 2016) which can easily be dismissed as just "feeling down," so it is vital to check your diet carefully for where you can get the vitamin.

Many people say that vegans suffer from iron problems due to their so-called lack of protein but Jessica Brown (2020) says this is mostly caused by not eating enough calories in the diet or making use of different colored fruits and vegetables in the diet. Lastly, consumption of legumes and pulses—seeds of legumes—can lead to problems with digestion as some people may find that they become bloated when eating this food source.

If one does not make up for what is lacking in a diet, then one is sure to fail or worse, get seriously ill. Luckily, folate—also known as folic acid—vitamin B12, calcium, and omega fatty acids can and should be supplemented. Vitamin B12 can be consumed through fortified foods—such as fortified cereals—or supplemented with either a monthly shot or daily pills. Calcium, folate, and omega fatty acids can all be bought in pill form from a pharmacy. If you find that your iron is lower than what you are comfortable with, then you can also supplement this with a pill or shot.

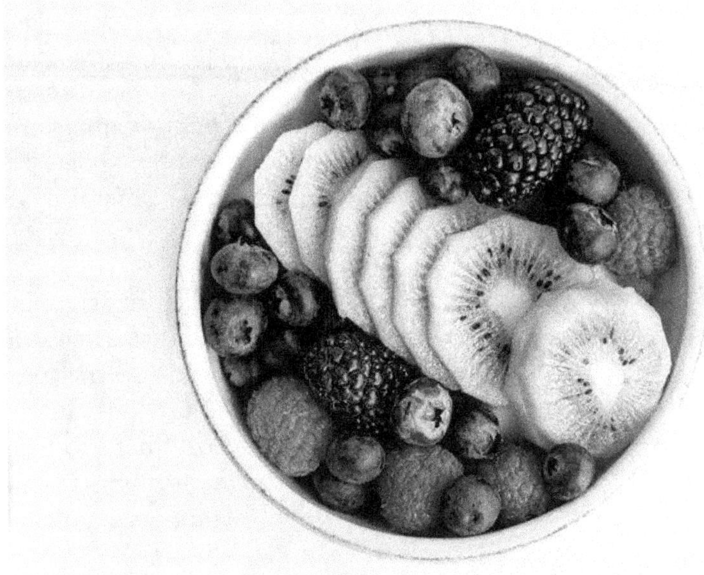

Duration

As being vegan is so much more than just a diet, there is no end date for being on this kind of eating pattern. There is only a starting date. This is a lifestyle where you will need to change many things about yourself to be fully immersed in it. There is also a cultural aspect of this lifestyle that not everyone will understand. Because of this, there may be judgment and many questions from people that simply cannot or will not understand why you may decide to take this route out of all other possible diets. The main thing to remember—and this is with every diet that will be discussed—change your diet because it is something you want or need, not because it is the "in thing" to do now. Not following the vegan diet carefully by keeping a careful eye on the vitamins and minerals you may need can be detrimental to your health.

Shopping List

Vegan isn't just about fruits and vegetables, so don't pause at the fresh section of your grocery store. To make sure you get all the calories, different fats, protein, carbohydrates, as well as the right vitamins and minerals, you will need to sit down and make a shopping list for yourself before going shopping. The only way to conquer a diet is to go into it fully prepared.

If you are someone who is making the change from a diet that contains animal products, perhaps consider gifting those items that remain in your fridge or pantry to people who do eat those products so that they do not go to waste. While you are removing the obvious animal products, take the time to go through the ingredients of other products you own to make sure you are not inadvertently consuming animal products. Watch out for words like lactose, whey, gelatin, casein, etc.

Many ingredients you will get from the shops can be used by other people, so if you share a home with non-vegans, this should not have too much of an impact on their diet. If you want to avoid eating from surfaces that have come into contact with animal products, then you should have your own cutting board, eating and preparation utensils, and perhaps your own level in the fridge and freezer. Many of the foods you will consume will be prepared fresh, so do not buy several months' worth of this as it will just go bad. Learn how to prepare variously cooked and uncooked plant-based foods and how to store them. Most cooked meals can last three to five days in the fridge but months in the freezer, either in its raw or cooked state.

Below you will find a shopping list put together by *Plenty Vegan* (2016), but it by no means covers all the possibilities that are available to you. This is but a guide. You will be in charge of making your own choices when it comes to filling that shopping cart, but it does give you a head start over those that don't have it.

- Fresh: All fruits, vegetables, and herbs

- Protein: Nuts, seeds, legumes, lentils, chickpeas, plant-based protein powders, tofu, tempeh, and any vegan suitable imitation meats, like Beyond Meat

- Vegan "dairy": Plant-based kinds of milk like coconut, rice, almond or soy, vegan cream cheese, vegan sour cream, vegan yogurt, vegan cheese

- Baking goods: Some baking goods may be vegan-friendly, but baking may need substitutes for eggs, butter, and milk.

- Fats: All plant-based fats such as olive oil, sunflower oil, and coconut oil

- Prepackaged goods: Here, you will need a skillful eye to make sure the ingredient list doesn't state any animal products. Avoid simply if not sure, as there could be possible cross contamination with animal products somewhere in the production.

- Grains: All grains are vegan-friendly as well as pasta in all forms but be wary of kinds of pasta that get stuffed, like ravioli.

- Snacks: Any dried fruit, popcorn you pop yourself, vegan chocolate, Oreos (be wary of cross contamination), and hard-boiled sweets that don't contain carmine (made from insects)

- Sauces: Hummus (made from chickpeas) and any that do not contain milk

There is a lot of debate surrounding the use of honey and eating figs when it comes to the vegan diet. Firstly, honey is produced by bees, usually on farms, and thus makes it an animal product, so it is not usually eaten by those on the vegan diet. The fig debate, however, is rather hotly contested by vegans, who some say it can be consumed while others say it can't be. Although the fig is plant-based, it is how it is pollinated that is causing a bit of a buzz. Figs do not have an external flower like other plants but an internal one that is pollinated by a wasp which has to crawl inside of the fruit to do so. The female does this to also lay her eggs in a safe place. The wasp later dies and remains inside the fruit to be dissolved as it grows (Petre, 2020). Some people believe because an animal has died to provide this fruit that it should not be consumed. However, a fig has no other way to be fertilized to provide seeds for future generations. So, on the other side of the coin, the relationship between wasp and fig is a beneficial one, and thus the insect has not been exploited, so the fruit can be consumed. At the end of the day, this is a choice you will have to make if you are someone who likes to eat figs.

Also, consider adding some supplements to your shopping list if you find yourself lacking in any of the nutrients discussed earlier.

Meal Plan

Now that you have chosen your specific vegan diet and completed your shopping, you will be able to start cooking delicious meals. If you have no recipes and don't simply want to just eat fruits and vegetables, have a look below for some examples of what you can eat. The below diet plan is for the plant-based vegan plan—where the emphasis is placed on plant-based foods and not calorie counting. If you want to try the other diets, then substitute what you want to eat for items that you do not like. The following meal plan was put together with the use of the works of Rachael Link (2019a) and Victoria Seaver (2019):

	Breakfast	Lunch	Dinner	Snacks
Day 1	Tempeh bacon with	Vegetable and hummus	Oat Risotto with spinach,	Bell peppers (all

	mushrooms, arugula, and avocado.	sandwich (one serving).	butternut squash, and mushrooms.	colors) with guacamole, seaweed chips, and fruit leather.
Day 2	Two vegan pancakes with ¼ cup blackberries, and a tablespoon of peanut butter.	One serving white bean & avocado toast with a cup sliced cucumber, seasoned with pepper and salt.	Mediterranean lentil salad with peppers (all colors), olives, cucumbers, kale, sun-dried tomatoes, and parsley.	Air-popped popcorn, trail mix, and kale chips.
Day 3	Coconut yogurt served with chia seeds, berries, and walnuts.	Four-cup serving of green salad with edamame and beets.	Cauliflower and chickpea tacos with pico de gallo (tomato and onion salsa) and guacamole.	One small plum and ¾ cup edamame pods, seasoned with salt and pepper.
Day 4	Sweet potato toast with peanut butter and topped with slices of banana.	Four-cup serving of white bean and vegetable salad.	Mushroom and lentil loaf with garlic, green beans, and cauliflower.	Pistachios, homemade muesli, and coconut chia pudding.

Day 5	Eggless quiche with silken tofu, broccoli, spinach, and tomatoes.	Whole grain pasta with meatballs made with lentils and a green salad.	Two cups of black-bean quinoa Buddha bowl.	Two tablespoons of pumpkin seeds and two cups of air-popped popcorn.
Day 6	Peanut butter-banana toast (one serving).	Tempeh taco salad with beans, quinoa, tomatoes, avocados, onions, and cilantro.	Falafel salad with lemon-tahini dressing (one serving).	½ cup of edamame pods, seasoned with spices.
Day 7	Peanut butter & chia berry jam English muffin (one serving).	Baked tofu with Brussels sprouts, red cabbage, and flavored couscous.	1 ½ cups of roasted cauliflower and potato curry soup with ½ a small whole wheat pita (toasted) and ⅓ cup hummus.	Mixed berries, walnuts, and a vegan protein shake.

Avoid making use of too many processed meals and stick to creating your own unique, homemade meals where you can. It is better for your health in the long run.

Chapter 2:

Vegetarian Diet

What Is It?

This diet is less restrictive than the vegan diet, as you are allowed to make use of some but not all animal products. This can also be treated as a lifestyle and not just a diet. Animal products that may be used include food items such as eggs and milk and clothing items such as wool. Similar to the vegan diet—which in itself is also a type of vegetarian diet—there are many kinds of vegetarian diets that you can make use of if you prefer a less restrictive diet. There are several types of vegetarians (Marcin, 2019; McPhillips, 2020):

- Lacto-ovo-vegetarian: A person that only eats dairy and egg supplied by animals, the classic vegetarian.

- Lacto-vegetarian: Someone who only eats dairy supplied by animals.

- Ovo-vegetarian: Someone who only eats eggs from animals.

- Vegetarian: A term used for someone who doesn't eat meat but is willing to make use of some animal products such as gelatin or collagen.

- Flexitarian: A term for a person who mostly eats plant-based but is willing to occasionally have a meat dish; semi-vegetarian.

- Pescatarian: A person who will still eat fish products, usually with the aim to become a lacto-ovo-vegetarian after some time.

- Pollo-vegetarians: Similar to the pescatarian, although these people make use of poultry in their diet and no other meat.

People who consider themselves "true" vegetarians will not consume any animal meat, but some people find it easier than others to make the switch to a new diet. Take the time to get familiar with each of the vegetarian diets before choosing which one you would like to follow. Many people switch to this diet for the same reasons as those who follow the vegan diet, while others just no longer want to eat meat.

Who Can Benefit?

Anyone can benefit from this lifestyle and diet change which has a little more freedom in terms of what one can eat when compared to a vegan diet. Depending on which kind of vegetarian diet you would like to follow, there are fewer items you will need to cut from your current diet. It is important to continue reading your ingredient labels, especially if you do not want to make use of any animal derivatives such as collagen, which can be found in some protein powders.

Pros

The advantages of a vegetarian diet are very similar to those found on the vegan diet (Link, 2018; Brazier, 2020a; Down to Earth, 2020). One's weight can be more easily managed—which helps fight obesity—as well as a decrease in cholesterol and various heart diseases. The diet offers some protection from certain cancers as well as lowering the chances of getting type 2 diabetes by stabilizing the blood sugar with the use of fiber. As one is living healthier, there is even an increase in the lifespan which is great news for those of us that want to live longer. This is because many plants contain not just fiber but also phytonutrients and antioxidants, which in turn help to strengthen the immune system and slow down the aging process. Because you are lowering your cholesterol and filling yourself up with healthy, high-fiber foods, you will find that your energy is showing an upward trend (Vegetarian Times Editors, 2007). More fiber is also great in that you will become more regular with your bowel movements while avoiding nasty hemorrhoids.

Your bones will be stronger than those on the vegan diet as you will be consuming more calcium if you are a lacto-ovo or lacto-vegetarian. The chance of coming into contact with foodborne diseases is also significantly lower on this diet than on a regular diet. With low-fat and high-fiber, a vegetarian diet is perfect for someone who may be suffering from menopause to help keep the extra pounds down due to a slowed metabolism. And, best of all, your plate is never boring and without color! Being on a vegetarian diet may also have an influence on improving symptoms of asthma sufferers (Marcin, 2019).

Cons

Similar to vegan diets, there are concerns about increased strokes happening while making use of the vegetarian diet (Doheny, 2019). Other concerns have been raised about brain health, as this diet is low in choline which is an essential nutrient our body needs. Though that said, vegetarians that make use of eggs do not have problems with choline. If a vegetarian is not strict on monitoring their protein intake, they may have hair loss. This is often seen in severe protein-deficient vegetarians.

There are also nutrient deficiencies in terms of omega-3 fatty acids, calcium—especially those that do not make use of milk—zinc, vitamin B12, and D (Frey, 2020c). However, if a person takes the time to look at the nutritional value of the foods consumed, then they can make use of supplements to fill in for what is missing in the diet. This does make the diet a little inconvenient as labels need to be checked not only for the nutrients but any possible animal products that one may not want to consume, as this will change depending on what kind of vegetarian you are.

As a vegetarian you are limited on the types of food you can and can't eat, so this can lead to boring meals if you are not creative in your cooking. Many of the food types one consumes on a vegetarian diet doesn't always make one feel full for an extended period. Because of this, there may be excessive snacking which can be detrimental to one's weight. This brings us to the point of vegetarian food, especially prepackaged foods, in that they may not always be so healthy, as there may be added fats and sugars that would normally not be there if you were to prepare your own food. Lastly, there is a concern that vegetarians may, in fact, be consuming more pesticides and herbicides than those that consume an omnivorous diet because of the increased plant foods that are eaten. This is why it is so important to wash *all* produce before making use of it.

Eating out can also be challenging, irrespective of which type of vegetarian you are because of the possibility of cross contamination with other food types that may be seen as undesirable by the consumer. Unless you know and trust the places you go out to eat at, perhaps give this a skip if you are concerned about this. The diet is harder to manage in terms of obtaining the nutrients needed, but luckily, one can use supplements to counteract this negative.

Duration

Vegetarianism is a lifestyle and not just a diet. You can remain on this diet for as long or as short as you want. The most important part is to choose which diet you will follow and then a starting point. Carefully go over foods you will need to make use of, and see where you may need to supplement, either through a change in the diet or by purchasing supplements from a pharmacy. Take the time to find restaurants that are well-known to the vegetarian community, and test them out for yourself.

If going full vegetarian is too difficult for you, consider becoming a semi-vegetarian where you increase your plant foods while slowly cutting meat out of your diet until you are comfortable with leaving it completely behind. Ensure that you have a vegetarian cooking only spot in your kitchen if you are concerned about cross contamination with another person's meals. If you have a child that has decided to become a vegetarian and you struggle to cook multiple different meals every day, then consider teaching the child to cook their meals or make use of premade vegetables or frozen vegetables instead of cleaning fresh veggies every day. Even an omnivore can stand a plant-based meal once a week and there are millions of interesting recipes online to be enticed by.

Shopping List

Each vegetarian diet type will have its unique shopping list due to its diet requirements. For the purpose of this list, the foods represented below will be for those that are completely vegetarian and make no use of animal meat at all. Some foods may still contain animal derivatives such as casein, gelatin, collagen, etc. If you are planning on sticking to a strict vegetarian diet where you need to cut out certain animal-based foods, it is strongly recommended that you read all the labels of your food before adding it to your cart. The list below was put together with information from *Plenty Vegan* (2016) as well as the research from Rachael Link (2018) and Yvette Brazier (2020a):

- Fresh: Many different fruits and vegetables, no limitations; similar to the vegan diet

- Protein: Nuts, seeds, eggs, legumes, pulses, plant-based protein powders, tofu, tempeh, and any imitation meats

- Dairy: Milk, yogurt, ice cream, cheese, cream cheese (only for lacto-ovo-vegetarians)

- Baking goods: All baked goods are vegetarian-friendly unless you are an ovo-vegetarian.

- Fats: All plant-based fats, no animal fats at all; similar to the vegan diet

- Prepackaged goods: Read labels carefully to avoid animal by-products.

- Grains: All grains are vegetarian-friendly, but whole grains are better than refined.

- Snacks: As long as the snack doesn't contain animal by-products you do not wish to consume, then enjoy.

- Sauces and soups: As long as the animal by-product of choice is avoided, most soups and sauces are fine.

- Other animal products: Honey (safe for all vegetarians)

For those that want to start the diet as semi-vegetarians, then buy fewer animal-based products every week and replace them with vegetarian-friendly items. Stick to lean, white meats to help you achieve this.

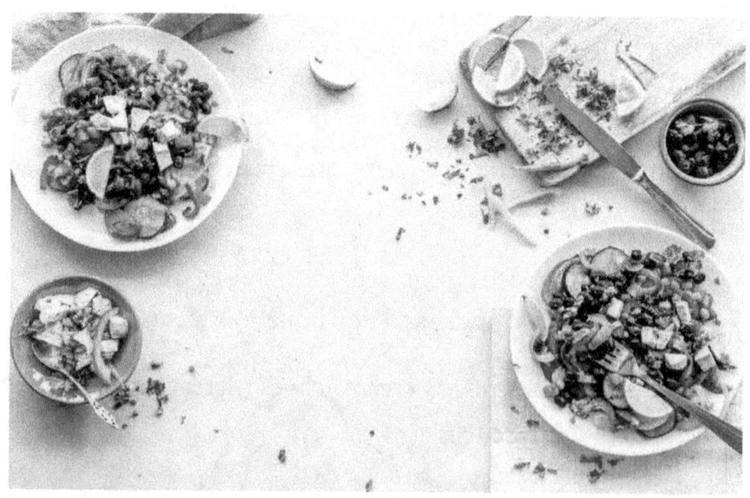

Similar to the vegan diet, learn to prepare and store fresh fruits and vegetables to limit the amount you will need to throw away due to spoilage. Consider buying fresh foods once a week while those that can be stored in a frozen form once a month. Only add supplements if required or directed so by a medical professional.

Meal Plan

As there are several vegetarian diets one can follow there, are multiple meal plans one can sit down and design for their own specific needs. The meal plans represented below are aimed at those that are the classic vegetarian (lacto-ovo-vegetarian), but if you are any other type of vegetarian, then you can simply remove which you do not want to eat, and supplement your food that abides by your dietary constraints. This meal plan was designed with the works of Rachael Link (2018), Rebecca Strong (2020), and Katie Bandurski (2021), with no concentration placed on the number of calories:

	Breakfast	Lunch	Dinner	Snacks
Day 1	Oatmeal, seasonal fruit, and flax seeds.	Roasted sweet potato & chickpea pitas with a small green salad.	Spicy peanut lettuce wraps with baked tofu, roasted peppers, cauliflower, and carrots with raw cucumbers.	Dried fruit and nut mix.

Day 2	Yogurt parfait with berries, muesli, and almonds.	Grilled veggie and hummus wrap with sweet potato fries.	Pepper ricotta primavera.	Vegetable sticks of choice with hummus or mayonnaise dip.
Day 3	Oatmeal waffles with cream or yogurt and fruit of choice topping.	Lentil soup and two slices of whole wheat bread.	Tofu banh mi sandwich with pickled vegetables.	Broccoli & chive-stuffed mini peppers.
Day 4	Powerhouse protein parfaits.	Red lentil veggie burger with a salad of choice.	Black bean burrito with a green salad.	Fruit and vegetable of choice smoothie.
Day 5	Two slices of whole wheat toast with ½ avocado.	Mediterranean bulgur bowl.	Garden-fresh grilled vegetable pizza.	Sliced apples with peanut butter and some sunflower seeds.
Day 6	Overnight baked eggs Bruschetta.	Large bowl with couscous, greens, vegetables (roasted or raw), drizzled in preferred dressing.	Vegetarian chili with some tortilla chips.	Roasted beetroot and garlic hummus with preferred raw vegetable sticks.

Day 7	Portobello mushrooms Florentine with one to two slices of whole wheat bread.	Arborio rice and white bean soup.	Vegetarian lasagna with a side plate of salad of choice; olive oil as dressing.	Crunchy roasted fava beans; try for salt-free if possible.

Regular cow's milk can be traded for almond or soy milk while eggs can be traded for silken tofu that can mimic scrambled eggs. Your imagination is the limit on this diet. When possible, avoid too many oils and processed foods. Ensure that your plate is always colorful and bursting with flavor. If you feel that you are still hungry add a few extra pieces of fruit to your snacking section.

Chapter 3:

Ketogenic Diet

What Is It?

The ketogenic diet—also known as the keto diet—is a diet that causes your body to use a different path of metabolism than it usually makes use of. In the previous two diets, the main source of energy came from carbohydrates in the form of mostly fruits and vegetables. Carbohydrates are broken down into various sugars and fibers upon digestion. The sugars, which can be simple or complex, are absorbed into the body where the glucose (blood sugar) is used to power the body as fuel. This metabolism is called glycolysis, and it is the body's go-to metabolism. When one is on the keto diet the main source of energy is not carbohydrates but rather fat. By limiting the body's access to glucose, by eating large quantities of fat, the body is forced to find an alternative metabolism to fuel itself. This is called ketosis (Editor, 2019). Ketosis is the metabolic process of breaking down fat into ketones which the body will then use as a new fuel source. The structure of a typical keto diet is high in fat, moderate in protein, and low to very low carbohydrates. There are several types of keto diets available:

- The standard keto diet (SKD): 70–80% fat, 15–20% protein, and 5–10% carbohydrates. The main idea is to keep the carbohydrates to between 20–50 grams a day.

- MCT keto diet: Sometimes it is difficult to consume large quantities of fats, so on this diet, the fats are supplemented by taking medium-chain triglycerides (MCT) to increase the fat content of the diet.

- Calorie-restricted keto diet: Usually keto diets are not calorie-restrictive due to the fat-burning properties, but if needed, you can limit the number of calories consumed on this diet.

- The cyclical keto diet (CKD): This diet seeks to add one to two days of carbohydrate-fueled days followed by five to six days on the SKD to build up the glycogen stores in the muscles. Normally reserved for people who exercise often.

- The targeted keto diet (TKD): Another diet targets those that like to work out. A small carbohydrate-heavy meal is consumed up to 30 minutes before a high-intensity training session.

- The high protein keto diet (HPKD): This is a diet more appropriate to those that want to build muscle than just losing weight. The protein content of the diet should be around 30–35% of the diet, 5% for carbohydrates, and the rest is made up of fat.

This is also a restrictive diet because you will need to keep a very close eye on your carbohydrate intake—the only way this diet will work for you is if you stay in ketosis and not go back to glycolysis. This is a tough diet to manage, but with a little planning and preparing, your food will become easier with time.

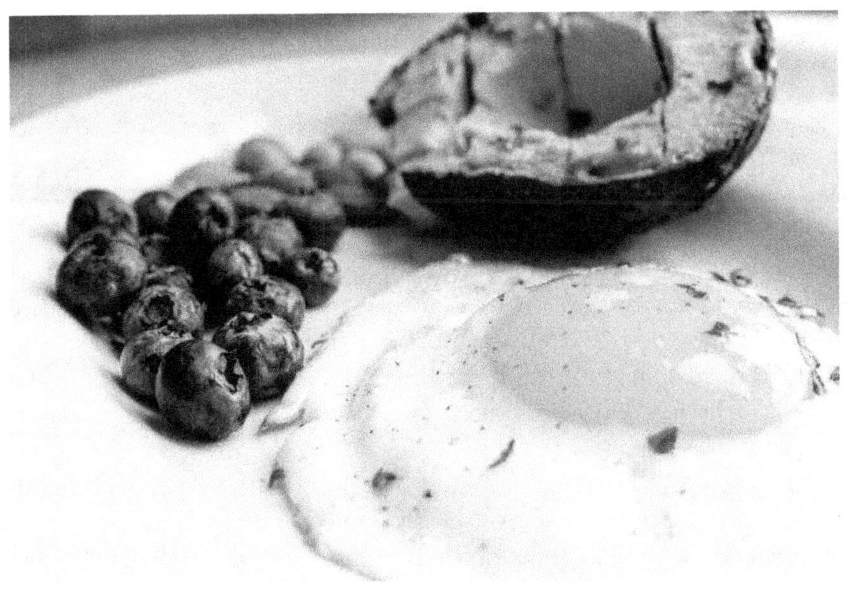

Who Can Benefit?

Although it is called a ketogenic diet, it isn't just a diet change but a complete lifestyle change. Due to the restrictive nature of this diet, those that love snacking on sweets, cakes, and sweet drinks may find this diet very difficult to start and follow through with. This is due to sugary goods having addictive properties, as it tends to trigger the pleasure centers of our brain (Hartney, 2020). This is why most people fail in their diets, irrespective of which one you follow. However, that said, this is the perfect diet to help people overcome their addiction to sugar, as all the foods that contain high levels of sugar cannot be eaten on this diet. Even the cravings for sugar, and carbohydrates in general, will fade as time progresses on the diet.

Pros

There are several advantages to one's health if one were to follow any of the ketogenic diets. The keto diet was one of the first diets to be used in treating seizures for those who suffered from epilepsy (Satterthwaite, 2018). It can also be used to manage type 2 diabetes as glucose is now used sparingly by the body, though it is a good idea to work together with a dietitian before just going off any medication. Not only is glucose being controlled, your insulin becomes more sensitive to reacting to it and stores it as glycogen in the muscles (The Portland Clinic, 2020). This diet is perfect for those seeking a way to cut all processed foods from their diet. With the higher consumption of fat, you will also feel satiated for longer than on any of the previously mentioned diets. As ketosis is the burning of fat for fuel, the loss of weight can be quite quick on this diet (Marshall, 2018). It is perfect for someone who has a low activity lifestyle and doesn't need the boost of energy that is required for exercise. Keto diets are also known for their cancer-fighting abilities as many cancer cells make use of glucose to develop. No glucose means that cancer cells grow far slower and can even become starved of the fuel they need to develop further.

The last advantage is the fact that you no longer have to worry about checking any food source to make sure it is fat-free (Northwestern Medicine Staff, 2019). You need the fat on this diet, but make sure you consume the healthier fats or your health will suffer.

Cons

It is believed that there is a risk of heart problems on this diet if too many saturated fats are consumed (Marshall, 2018) in favor of unsaturated fats. Though that said, there is scientific research around saturated fats and heart problems where no significant evidence of problems was found (Hoenselaar, 2012; Nettleton et al., 2017). Though it must be noted that if one makes use of polyunsaturated fats in favor of saturated fats, there is an anti-inflammatory effect which in itself is great for one's health (Gunnars, 2018a).

If you are someone who prides themselves in the gym, you may find that this diet causes you to lose your edge. Unless you are making use of the CKD or the TKD, which allows for the extra consumption of carbohydrates, you may find you just do not have the energy to complete your usual workout. Although glucose is not bad, your body still needs it for certain bodily functions and organs, so cutting it out of your diet completely is not a good idea. Luckily, protein can undergo gluconeogenesis in the liver to produce glucose if the body needs it. This is why the keto diet calls for moderate protein.

Restrictive diets always come with problems in trying to maintain the correct nutritional balance, and as keto cuts back on a lot of fruits, vegetables, and grains, you will find you will be lacking in vitamins and fiber. This lack of fiber can lead to many stomach issues (Satterthwaite, 2018) which could either be constipation or diarrhea. Consider taking supplements to ease any discomfort or lack of nutrients.

Due to the shift in metabolism, a person is often left feeling tired, having headaches, nausea, and even cravings for treats you have been forced to give up. This is known as keto flu and it feels as bad as having the flu. However, this is a temporary state that will get better once you are fully in ketosis. Frequent urination is also a side effect of the diet (Northwestern Medicine Staff, 2019). This is because glycogen is stored in the muscles with extra water, and once the glycogen is used up the water is free to be removed from the body. This not only causes dehydration but also a loss of essential salts which can lead to cramping of the muscles. People who have kidney problems shouldn't make use of this diet due to the ketones and protein waste that accompanies frequent urination.

People who suffer from obsessive-compulsive disorder (OCD) may become too extreme and focused on micromanaging this diet and may even result in an eating disorder. A way to alleviate this is to give them a balanced keto diet that is already worked out for their specific needs.

This way they do not need to become obsessed with having to check all their food all the time.

Duration

Once ketosis is reached and supplements are used to address the nutrient deficiencies, most of the disadvantages of this diet are more manageable or completely disappear. However, this diet is quite difficult to adhere to because of the negatives, and many people decide to quit before the real benefits are seen. Liz Satterthwaite (2018) states that 30 days is not enough to gain all the benefits from this diet, and one should consider a longer period to see if the diet suits you or not. The ketogenic diet can either be used as a diet or as a lifestyle change.

As great as the advantages are on this diet, it is difficult to maintain and requires a person to be vigilant in controlling their macromolecules (protein, fat, and carbohydrates). It is a good idea to make use of macromolecule calculator apps and websites that show what nutrients are in the foods you are preparing. *Diet Doctor* is a fantastic website that answers many questions and gives you access to a wide variety of recipes and articles. One needs to be willing to prepare meals well, while being aware of what goes into the production of the meal, and avoid all prepackaged meals.

Once you have built up your confidence while being on the diet, you can make use of your knowledge to decide where are the best places to eat. Any place that makes food that caters to the Atkins—to be discussed later—or paleo diet is perfect for a keto eater.

Shopping List

Although limited on vegetables, fruits, and grains, this diet allows for various meat and animal products while avoiding all processed foods where possible. Premade foods require you to check the label carefully to make sure that you remain within the budget of your keto diet type. If you want to make sure that you are getting the healthier options in terms of fats, don't be afraid to make use of plant-based fats which contain all the goodness that you may be missing. This shopping list was put together with the works of Andreas Eenfeldt (2021a; 2021b) and Franziska Spritzler (2021):

- Fresh: Fruits and vegetables eaten should be at no more than 10 grams net carbs per 3.5 ounces. Below are the fresh fruits and vegetables from the lowest amount of net carbohydrates to the highest:

  - Fruit: Raspberries, blackberries, strawberries, cantaloupe, peach, clementine, cherries, and plums; Blueberries can be made use of but they are 12 grams net carbs per 3.5 ounces serving, so use sparingly.

  - Vegetables: Spinach, olives, asparagus, tomatoes, avocado, kale, lettuce, zucchini, cauliflower, eggplant, cabbage, Brussels sprouts, broccoli, cucumber, green beans, and peppers are all under five grams net carbs. Those that are a little higher in carbohydrates but under 10 grams net include rutabaga, onion, carrot, celeriac, and beets.

- Protein: Nuts, seeds, eggs, protein powders, tofu, tempeh, and any type of meat, but be wary of processed meats like sausage or bacon.

- Dairy: All dairy is allowed but used moderately as some dairy, like milk, contains lactose which is milk sugar. Butter, ghee, and cheese are the go-to snacks on this diet.

- Baking goods: Prebaked goods are a no-no because they contain grains that are too high in carbohydrates, but you can make use of almond and coconut flour as there are keto-friendly recipes available. Use keto-friendly sweeteners to replace sugar.

- Fats: All fats are usable but they make use of the healthiest unsaturated fats to protect your heart—lard, tallow, coconut oil, avocado oil, etc.

- Prepackaged goods: Read labels carefully to avoid carbohydrates or avoid completely.

- Grains: Zero grains are allowed on this diet.

- Snacks: Unless you are making your own, it is best to avoid store-bought.

- Sauces and soups: Avoid the canned kind and make your own. Bone broth is wonderful to replace any nutrients you may be lacking.

If you are a vegan that wants to try a keto diet, it is very possible, just avoid the animal products. However, your diet becomes very restrictive which can lead to even more nutrient deficiencies in your diet. While on the keto diet, many foods that you can no longer eat can be replaced with those that you can. An example is French fries. You cannot eat starchy vegetables at all on a keto diet but if you take celeriac—the root of the celery plant—and you cut it into strips, you can deep fry them to get the same texture as French fries. This diet does require a little practice and creativity.

Meal Plans

A keto diet can be as restrictive as what your imagination allows it to be. Getting the high level of fat required can be a tough chore, but make use of MCT supplements as well as many plant-based oils to go with your salads as well as your cooking. For the following meal plan, only the standard keto diet will be represented. If you want to make use of the high-protein keto diet, you can simply add more protein while lowering the amount of fat you eat. If you are interested in making use of the targeted keto diet then eat a small bowl of white rice or pasta before training, though this is only suggested for people who are training moderately most of the week. When trying the cyclical keto diet, eat a majority of healthy carbohydrates over fat during your non-keto day(s) before returning to the keto diet you were on previously. This meal is made up of the works of Mellissa Sevigny (2014), *All Day I Dream About Food* (2020), and Andreas Eenfeldt (2021c):

	Breakfast	Lunch	Dinner	Snacks
Day 1	Keto-friendly sheet pan pancakes.	½ cup simple egg salad with lettuce leaves and two slices of cooked bacon.	Keto-friendly pesto chicken casserole with feta cheese and olives.	½ avocado with salt and pepper, or lemon juice to taste.
Day 2	Frittata with fresh spinach.	One cup of chopped chicken, two cups of chopping lettuce drizzled with two tablespoons Caesar salad dressing (sugar-free).	Chicken and broccoli casserole.	24 raw almonds.
Day 3	Dairy-free	Keto-friendly	Asian steak	Chocolate

	latte.	quesadillas.	bites.	and peanut butter chaffle.
Day 4	Two cream cheese pancakes with two pieces of cooked bacon followed by coffee with two tablespoons of heavy cream (or bulletproof coffee).	Mexican cauliflower rice.	Keto pizza, add meat of choice if more fat and protein is needed for the day.	One cup of bone broth, two string cheese packets.
Day 5	Cinnamon crunch cereal low-carb.	One Italian sausage link, cooked chopped up then add ¾ cup of easy cauliflower gratin.	Keto-friendly meat pie.	Fat bombs and bulletproof coffee if more fat is needed.
Day 6	Egg and bacon casserole.	Bacon, avocado, and goat cheese salad.	Sheet pan chicken, and vegetables, always choose low-carb veggies where you can.	Keto butter pecan cookies.

| Day 7 | Keto-friendly pancakes with berries, and whipped cream. | 1 ½ cup of Chili spaghetti squash casserole. | 1 cup Cuban pot roast on top of two cups chopped lettuce. Mixture topped with two tbsp of sour cream and ¼ cup of grated, sharp cheddar cheese. | Two squares Lindt 90% chocolate. |

If you are finding yourself getting hungry despite the meal plan, then consider adding more fat to your diet. This can be through supplements or by using fattier cuts of meat. If you are a vegetarian—if vegan, you will have to cut out all animal products—that would like to try a keto diet, then try the following meal plan that was put together with the works of Martina Slajerova (2019), Rachael Link (2019b), and Craig Clarke (2020):

	Breakfast	Lunch	Dinner	Snacks
Day 1	Chocolate Smoothie.	Garlic and herb mock monkey bread.	"Tricolore" salad (add extra coconut or olive oil over the top if you need the fat).	Low-carb coconut chip cookies.
Day 2	Two-egg omelet made with coconut	Egg stuffed avocado.	Fried cauliflower rice made with	Tropical chocolate mousse

	oil, onions, cheese, tomatoes, and add salt and pepper to taste.		coconut oil, low-carb vegetables, and crispy tofu.	bites.
Day 3	Pumpkin spice French toast.	Cauliflower mac and cheese with mock bacon, avocado oil, and broccoli.	Egg muffins (three portions).	Keto vanilla bean cupcakes.
Day 4	Frittata with cheese and tomatoes.	Cauliflower-crust pizza with cheese, diced tomatoes, mushrooms, some olive oil, and spinach or kale.	Zucchini pizza boats made with olive oil and stuffed with keto-friendly marinara, spinach cheese, and garlic.	Vegetarian fat bombs.
Day 5	Tofu scramble with olive oil, mixed with low-carb vegetables, and cheese.	Grilled vegetable and fried goat cheese salad.	Vegetarian lasagna.	Low-carb vegetables with keto-friendly dip.
Day 6	Buttermilk pancakes can be topped	Avocado and egg salad.	A salad made with flavored greens and	Boiled eggs with sour cream.

	with whipped heavy cream and berries.		topped with crispy tofu, avocados, tomatoes, and bell peppers (green).	
Day 7	Smoothie prepared with full-fat milk, spinach, peanut butter, MCT oil, and chocolate whey protein powder (vegetarian friendly).	Taco lettuce wraps with avocados, walnut-mushroom meat, tomatoes, sour cream, cheese, and cilantro.	Zucchini with avocado and walnut pesto.	Keto cookies and crème ice cream.

If you come across any vegetarian recipes that call for mock bacon—bacon not from an animal source—make use of these recipes to make your own bacon:

- Vegan bacon using tofu.
- Vegan bacon using mushrooms (Use low-carb maple syrup to keep it keto-friendly.)

Irrespective of whether you are vegetarian, vegan, or an omnivore, remember to keep your carbohydrates low and your fat high with the aid of a macromolecule calculator. The way to be successful on a keto diet is to prepare your meals in advance knowing exactly what is in them. Make use of many resources to find recipes that best suit your diet.

Chapter 4:

Atkins Diet

What Is It?

The Atkins diet is very similar to the keto diet due to it also being a low carbohydrate diet (Gunnars, 2018c). It is also a restrictive diet where you will need to give up a lot of processed foods as well as many sugary and starchy items. However, where it differs from the keto diet is that the Atkins diet allows for the addition of healthy carbohydrates later in the diet. When one is eating fewer carbs and making use of more protein and fat, you will feel full much longer, and thus causes you to eat less food and naturally restrict your amount of calories you consume.

There are four phases to the full Atkins diet, although not everyone makes use of them if they have a well-balanced Atkins meal plan. Before starting this diet, it is a good idea to know what your goal weight is as this is needed for Phase Three of the diet. Below you can see the different phases:

- Introduction (Phase One): Follow a keto-like diet where you eat less than 20 grams of carbohydrates a day for two weeks. This phase is used to get the body into the fat-burning and weight-loss stage.

- Balancing (Phase Two): There is a slow addition of nuts as well as a small amount of low-carb fruit and more low-carb vegetables.

- Fine-Tuning (Phase Three): As you start to near your goal weight, continue to add more carbs to your diet. Your weight loss should start to slow down. Continue to make an effort to avoid all refined and processed foods.

- Maintenance (Phase Four): Continue to eat at the level of carbohydrates where your weight is being maintained at your ideal standard.

This diet is also suited to vegetarians and vegans with a little more planning around where the fats in the diet will come from. The way to beat a diet is research, so be sure to educate yourself if you are putting yourself on an already restrictive diet.

If one struggles with maintaining a keto lifestyle but doesn't want to lose the progress they have made, then switching to the Atkins diet is the perfect transition. It allows for the inclusion of different carbohydrates while still avoiding a lot of the foods which are considered too high in carbohydrates.

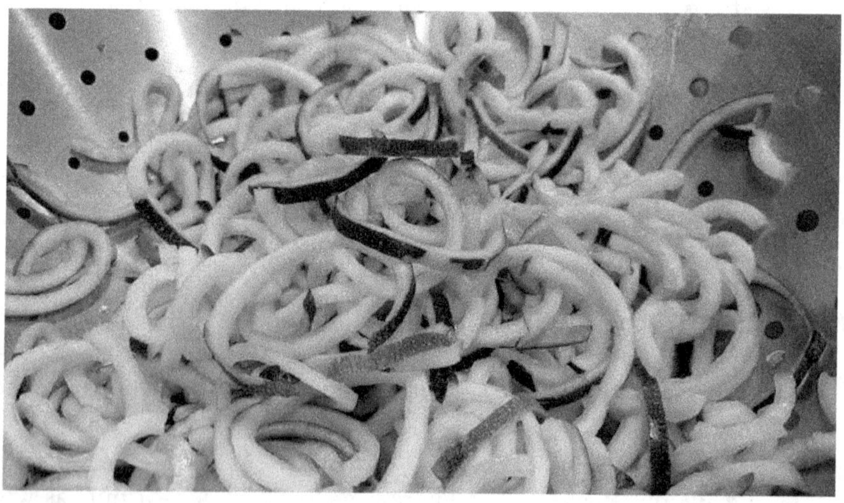

Who Can Benefit?

Although this diet starts very restrictive, similar to a ketogenic diet, it does ease the restriction after about two weeks. This diet is perfect for someone who wants to lose a set amount of weight and then maintain it. This diet is a great way to cut out food that is considered "junk" and heavy in refined sugars. It also encourages people to eat more fruits and vegetables which have various benefits.

Pros

The initial phase of this diet has similar advantages to the keto diet, with quite a lot of weight loss due to entering ketosis (Scott, 2020). This diet is fairly easy to follow, as there are guidelines to help reach the weight goals decided upon. That said, the diet is not strict on calorie counting but allows for the consumption of high protein and fat in the diet (Robertson, 2017). Although the protein content can be as high as 35%, this diet does not show any kidney stone development which can sometimes occur on the keto diet. With one being encouraged to eat fattier foods, it makes shopping a lot easier if you don't have to be on the lookout for items that state they are low in fat. Because of how well the Atkins diet has been researched, you will be able to find all manner of resources online or in print to help you with your journey.

The diet is not time-consuming and rather affordable (Better Health USA, 2007). With clear guidelines, you can shop for ingredients and foods that not only fit your budget but also your disappearing waistline. Unlike the keto diet, the later phases of Atkins allow for more carbohydrates to be added to the diet and thus allow for more variation when it comes to your food choices. Even in Phase One, the Atkins diet focuses on fiber-rich carbohydrates in the form of low-carb vegetables.

Cons

Phase one has the worst of the disadvantages of the Atkins diet (Scott, 2020). As you are forcing your body into ketosis—due to eating about 20 grams of carbs a day—you will suffer from keto flu. Side effects include but are not limited to dehydration, nausea, and hunger pangs. The initial start of the diet is very restrictive in fruits and grains which can lead to constipation. Not only that, but if you are a social butterfly, the diet will make it difficult to eat at most restaurants unless they serve low-carb meals.

As the first two weeks of this diet forces your body into ketosis, you will need to monitor your net carbohydrates—also known as digestible carbs—closely, for if you go above a certain amount, you will be kicked out of ketosis and lose the benefits of the fat-burning metabolic state. Because this time is so restrictive on the food you may eat, you may be faced with deficiencies and have to rely on supplements if there are any problems.

There will also be an increase in cholesterol levels (Robertson, 2017). This is where one needs to look at the whole cholesterol profile to determine what your true cholesterol is. Cholesterol is made up of three parts: high-density lipoprotein (HDL), low-density lipoprotein (LDL), and triglycerides. As long as the "good" cholesterol (HDL) is high and your "bad" cholesterol (LDL) is low, then your cholesterol is good. The HDL is the cholesterol that combats the other forms of cholesterol and removes it from your bloodstream (Mayo Clinic Staff, n.d.). Always look at the whole profile and not just the cholesterol to see where your problem may lie. The type of fat, trans fats, you consume can affect your heart (Better Health USA, 2007). Always make healthy fat choices and avoid all man-made fats such as trans fats which are not good for your health.

Duration

Although Phase One of the Atkins diet states that you shouldn't be on it longer than o two weeks, many people like to remain on it longer because of the rapid loss of weight (Sundblad, n.d.). In Phases Two and Three, there are no time limits at all and Phase Four is just about maintaining the weight you have decided upon.

If you can comfortably remain at Phase One then it is possible to make it a lifestyle choice, but then it is a keto lifestyle. The Atkins diet is about the loss of weight and then maintaining that weight. There is no time limit. So, in essence, as long as your body reacts well to the lower levels of carbohydrates, then you can maintain this lifestyle for as long as you are comfortable. If there is an increase in weight, then you can simply look at lowering the level of carbohydrates consumed, or switch to Phase One until the desired weight is reached once more.

Shopping List

This diet has different requirements of food as you progress through it so the shopping list will be divided into two parts. The first part will be aimed at Phase One and the second part will be for the remaining phases. These lists were created using the works of Kris Gunnars (2018c) and Atkins (n.d.-a, n.d.-b). For a more comprehensive list, visit the Atkins website where lists for each phase are available.

Introduction Shopping List

- Fresh: Vegetables that are eaten during the Introduction phase should be similar to the vegetables that are eaten on the keto diet. The lower the carbs, the better.

- o   Fruit: Avoid for the first two weeks, or make use of keto-friendly fruits.

  - o   Vegetables: All keto-friendly vegetables including alfalfa sprouts, radishes, Swiss chard, beet greens, portobello mushrooms, spaghetti squash, etc.

- Protein: No limit on meat; the fattier the better (unless vegan or vegetarian). Look to using full-fat tofu if trying this diet as a vegan or vegetarian or use a small portion of nuts.

- Dairy: Cheese, cream cheese, and cream; keep dairy products in moderation as they do contain carbs.

- Fats: All plant and animal-based fats

- Prepackaged goods: Avoid if at all possible, or follow the rules set out in the keto diet.

- Grains: Zero grains are allowed during this phase.

- Snacks: Keto-friendly while avoiding nuts in all forms

- Beverages: As long as they are low on carbohydrates, you can drink, though it is best to make use of broths and water if you are worried about the carbs accumulating.

Food to completely avoid during this step are your legumes, high-carb fruits, and vegetables, such as carrots or bananas, as well as your starchy vegetables, such as potatoes. These can be included in the later phases of the diet. If you are concerned about monitoring your net carbs, make use of a macromolecule app calculator. This will help you design your meals so that you know exactly how many carbohydrates you are putting into your body.

Remaining Phases Shopping List

If you find that you enjoy the foods from the first shopping list, then you may continue to eat them but do add a few more items to your shopping list to increase the variety of carbohydrates that you eat. Carbohydrates are not the enemy if you know how to control your eating habits. The following will not include anything that was already discussed in the previous list, as this list just builds on what you already have available to you.

- Fresh: Increase the number of vegetables and fruits that you can eat. Portion control is necessary due to the increase of carbohydrates associated with some of the fruits and vegetables. If possible, always go with the higher fiber option.

    o Fruits: All berries, cantaloupe, honeydew, watermelon, apple, cherry, plums, etc.

    o Vegetables: Beets, sweet corn, potatoes, butternut squash, etc.

- Protein: Nuts of all kinds, starting with small portions of about two tablespoons.

- Dairy: Yogurt, milk, and cottage cheese

- Legumes: Beans of all kinds (avoid baked beans), and chickpeas, about ¼ cup

- Grains: Start slow on grains; small portions (two tablespoons up to ½ a cup depending on grain) allowed from Phase Three

- Snacks: Keto-friendly or Atkins approved.

- Beverages: Avoid fruit juice or include water considerably.

One will still need to keep a close eye on the consumption of any carbohydrates, but there is more freedom when one moves over to the last phases of this diet.

Meal Plans

Two meal plans will be presented in this section. The first will be for Phase One and the second will be for the remainder of the diet. Once you have managed to complete Phase One, then make use of the next meal plan to help you control your weight loss and then maintain it for however long you want to. If you feel you are picking up too much weight again after several weeks at Phase Four, then you can lower the number of carbohydrates you eat to see if this helps.

Introduction Diet (Phase One)

The meal plan for Phase One was put together with the works of Atkins (n.d.-c; n.d.-d) and Karen Spaeder (2019):

	Breakfast	Lunch	Dinner	Snacks
Day 1	Two-egg omelet stuffed with ¼ cup favored cheese and ½ cup sliced green pepper.	Lean beef stir fry with red onion, broccoli, and bok choy.	½ cup ground beef cooked with ½ cup tinned tomatoes (low sugar) with ½ onion. Serve in lettuce leaves with two tbsp	½ tin tuna with full-fat mayonnaise (low-sugar) on a lettuce leaf, add ¼ cup cubed cheese of choice.

Day			guacamole. Season to taste.	
Day 2	Spinach or kale and cheese omelet topped with homemade salsa, and sliced avocado.	A grilled chicken thigh served with mixed greens, ½ chopped green pepper, a few cucumber slices, and ½ of favored cheese.	Grilled chicken and low-carb vegetable kabobs.	A boiled egg and eight olives.
Day 3	3.5 ounces smoked salmon with ½ an avocado and two tablespoons cream cheese, sprinkle with black pepper for taste.	Chicken or turkey meatballs served over spaghetti squash.	A slice of baked pork belly served with ⅔ cup of broccoli and cauliflower mashed with one tablespoon butter. Add ½ cup grated cheese of choice.	Cherry tomatoes with cream cheese, and cucumber slices with sour cream.
Day 4	Two eggs with bacon and ½ cup of low-carb vegetables.	A can of mackerel or tuna (in brine), served with 3 ½ cups spinach, crumble ½	Ground turkey taco salad with low-carb vegetables and an ounce of grated cheddar cheese.	One pepperoni stick and ½ mashed avocado spread into celery.

		cup of feta, and ½ chopped green pepper over the top.		
Day 5	Two poached eggs with 1 ¼ cups mushrooms and two strips bacon cooked in coconut oil sprinkle. Add parsley, salt, and pepper to taste.	Mixed green salad topped with diced raw low-carb vegetables and grilled chicken.	Two smoky chorizo sausages served with ⅔ cup cauliflower, cooked and mashed together with one tbsp cream cheese, and ½ cup green beans.	¼ avocado and one slice of cheese rolled in a lettuce leaf with ½ cup cubed cheese of choice.
Day 6	One egg fried in a tablespoon coconut oil, one low carb sausage, and grilled mushrooms.	Grill two tomato halves, top with ½ cup mozzarella cheese, two slices turkey, drizzle with a tablespoon olive oil and a teaspoon balsamic vinegar for flavor.	Ground beef burger served on lettuce with ½ cup low-carb vegetables.	A slice of ham and cheese wrapped together and a cooked chicken leg.

| Day 7 | Loaded low-carb vegetable two-egg omelet. | One burger (no bread) topped with ½ sliced avocado and a small tomato. Add a green salad drizzled with olive oil. | A chicken breast wrapped in two slices of prosciutto. Serve together with 3.5 ounces celeriac (celery root) mashed with a tablespoon of butter. | Two tablespoons cream cheese spread into some celery stalks and ½ an avocado. |

Remember to check Phase One's shopping list to see what your low-carb vegetables are before you start cooking. You should follow Phase One for two weeks before moving onto Phase Two. You can either repeat the above diet twice, or you can make use of the ketogenic diet in the previous chapter, or design your own week-long meal plan with the shopping list above.

Remainder of Diet

This is the first week of the Balancing Phase where you can eat up to about 25 g of carbohydrates. As the remaining phases (Fine Tuning and Maintenance Phases) progress, you can add more and more carbohydrates until you are happy with where you are in the diet. Always choose to eat healthy carbohydrates and avoid making use of processed and refined products where you can. The meal plan below was designed using the works of Atkins (n.d.-e; n.d.-f):

	Breakfast	Lunch	Dinner	Snacks
Day 1	One cup full-fat plain	A tin salmon served with a	Two low-carb sausages with	¼ cup hazelnuts

	Greek yogurt with three tablespoons three tablespoons of blueberries (fresh or frozen).	small mixed green salad, ½ chopped red pepper, some cucumber slices, and four radishes. Add a tablespoon full-fat mayonnaise (sugar-free) and top with ½ cup cheese of choice.	cauliflower mash made with full-fat cream cheese topped with grated cheddar with green beans on the side.	and five strawberries with two tablespoons cream.
Day 2	Two strips of bacon with sliced tomato, ½ cup grated cheese of choice, and fried mushrooms.	Mix a can of tuna with a tablespoon of mayonnaise then add some chopped celery, olives, and cherry tomatoes. As a side dish, have one cup full-fat plain Greek yogurt topped with three tablespoons of raspberries.	Grill half of a lamb steak and serve with ⅔ cup steamed cauliflower with a cheese sauce and some dark green vegetables that were sautéed in oil. Add a side dish of two slices of cantaloupe.	Two tbsp hummus with chopped red or green pepper strips and ½ cup cottage cheese mixed with three tablespoons of blueberries.

Day 3	Two poached eggs topped with two strips of bacon with sautéed (using a tbsp of coconut oil) mushrooms, and ½ grilled tomato.	A can of tuna (in brine) served with 3 ½ cups spinach, ½ cup crumbled feta, ½ chopped green pepper, some chopped radishes, with a drizzle with olive oil.	One large pork chop, topped with mustard then grilled. Serve on a bed of 3 ½ cups kale, cooked in one tablespoon butter, and 1 ¼ cups steamed Brussels sprouts.	10 green olives and ¼ cup hazelnuts.
Day 4	One cup full-fat plain Greek yogurt topped with a handful of shaved almonds and three tablespoons berry of choice.	A can of tuna mixed with a tablespoon full-fat (sugar-free) mayonnaise. Serve with a small green salad with five cherry tomatoes, five black olives, ⅓ red pepper, and three chopped radishes.	4 oz cod serving baked in tin foil, topped with a tbsp butter and a tsp parsley. Serve with 2 ½ cups "riced" cauliflower and buttered 1 ¼ cups Brussels sprouts.	Two tablespoons full-fat cream cheese spread into a celery stalk and ¼ cup almonds.

Day 5	Two-egg omelet filled with ½ cup grated cheese of choice with ½ an avocado and ½ grilled tomato.	Kebabs made with ¾ cup cubed chicken breast, ½ cubed green pepper, some mushrooms, and ⅓ red onion served with side green salad. On a side plate have two slices of cantaloupe with ½ cup cottage cheese.	Grill one beef burger (no bread), with ½ avocado and ½ cup of feta. All served on lettuce leaves with a large mixed salad (low-carb) and celeriac chips.	One carrot cut into sticks with a dip of two tbsp full-fat cream cheese and ¼ cup strawberries.
Day 6	One cup full-fat plain Greek yogurt two tablespoons almond shavings and two tablespoons raspberries.	A chicken breast mixed with ¼ cup, chorizo, and chopped tomatoes. Allow to simmer for 40 minutes and serve with kale and sugar peas.	Chicken breast stuffed with ¼ cup ricotta cheese and wrapped in ham. Serve with 3 ½ cups spinach and ¼ cup pine nuts, cooked in olive oil.	A handful of mixed nuts, with two tablespoons hummus with one chopped carrot.
Day	Two-egg	Slice ½ cup of	Flatten a	½ can tuna

7	omelet filled with mushrooms sautéed in olive oil, add ½ cup cheese of choice and chopped spring onion.	mozzarella and place on top of sliced tomato, top this with shredded basil leaves, and drizzle with a tablespoon of olive oil.	chicken breast then fill with 3 ½ cups slightly wilted spinach and ½ cup of ricotta cheese then wrap in two slices of prosciutto. Serve together with a cup of celeriac mash made with a tablespoon of butter.	with full-fat (sugar-free) mayonnaise using lettuce as a wrap. Make guacamole by adding ½ an avocado, one chopped spring onion, and two diced cherry tomatoes. Add to wrap.

Add low-carb fruit to the diet after a week following Phase Two until you reach Phase Four. If you decide after some time at Phase Four that you would like to lose more weight, you can transition back to Phase One and continue until you are close to your goal weight. Then follow the steps from there until you reach Phase Four again.

Chapter 5:

Low-Fat Diet

What Is It?

This diet is the opposite of what was discussed with the previous two diets. The low-fat diet—sometimes referred to as a low-cholesterol diet—seeks to remove as much fat from the diet as possible. This can be done by making dietary choices where high-fat foods are removed, low-fat meats are consumed, as well as fat being trimmed off of any meats (Drugs.com, 2020). The idea behind this diet is to restrict the number of fats you each which in turn will lower the number of calories you consume. Each gram of the macronutrients that we consume each gives us a certain amount of calories. A gram of fat yields nine calories, while a gram of carbohydrates and protein yields about four grams each (Gavin, 2018). Because of this, the more fat you eat, the more calories you consume, which in turn causes one to pick up weight (Dansinger, 2021). The fats that are generally targeted are unhealthy fats such as saturated fats, cholesterol, as well as trans fats such as shortening or margarine.

This diet requires the fat content to be between 20–35% of your total diet. So, if you are eating 2,000 kcal a day you need to be consuming between 44–77 grams of fat. Fat cannot be completely removed from the diet because without fat your health will suffer. Some vitamins—A, D, E, and K—are fat-soluble, so if there is no fat, you will not be able to make use of these vitamins (Yetman, 2020). You will also suffer dermatitis (skin irritations and rashes), a lower degree of healing from wounds, hair loss, as well as a weakened immune system causing you to fall ill frequently. So, even though fat needs to be kept low, there are plenty of fats you can make use of. If bad fats are unavoidable in your diet, then you will need to limit the amount you consume (Drugs.com, 2020):

- Trans fats: Avoid completely if possible; if not, eat less fried foods.

- Cholesterol: Try to keep below 200 mg per day.

- Saturated fat: No more than seven percent of your daily calories should be made up of this fat.

Healthier fat options come from plant sources, such as avocado oil, olive oil, etc., which should be consumed in higher dosages over animal-based fats. One should concentrate on only consuming monounsaturated and polyunsaturated fats. Many protein sources also have higher fat content in them, so it is a good idea to look for foods that contain the words low-fat—this is especially true for milk, cheese, yogurt, and even tofu—though be careful with some products that may be artificially sweetened after being made low-fat. Keep protein sources moderate and as lean as possible, making use of both animal-based and plant-based options.

Even though this diet is all about removing as many bad fat sources as possible, it is also important to count the number of calories you eat and control the number of carbohydrates you make use of daily. Being in a deficit through eating less and getting exercise makes this diet work at its best.

Spotting and dealing with fats in a diet can be a little tough but once you have the knack of the following you should be fine in avoiding those excess and unwanted calories (Reyzelman, 2017; Dansinger, 2021):

- Do not fry any food. Make use of grilling, baking, or even broiling your food on a rack so that the fat drips away from what you eat.

- Read the labels on everything you purchase to make sure of the fat content.

- Excess fat can be trimmed away from meat, and poultry can have the skin removed.

- Free-floating fat from stews can be scooped out once the dish is cooled, the same can be done for soups or broths.

- Instead of adding oils as flavorings to your vegetables and salads, try some lemon juice with various other spices and herbs.

- You do not need to remove your favorite meat, even if it is fattier than most. Simply cut the portion size and have it accompanied with several sides of high-fiber vegetables.

- Find replacements for your favorite cream toppings. Use plain yogurt with some green onions instead of sour cream as it will have less fat.

Who Can Benefit?

If you are unable to digest fats, i.e. not having a gallbladder, this is the perfect diet for you (Drugs.com, 2020). This is the kind of diet that helps to restrict calorie intake by avoiding the consumption of fats.

Pros

In terms of short-term weight loss, this is the ideal weight to make use of as long as the low level of fat in the diet is countered by well-balanced, nutrient-rich carbohydrates and good quality proteins

(Fogoros, 2021). It also works well for those that wish to simply maintain their weight (Rayzelman, 2017). A diet that is low in all the bad fats will cause one's cholesterol to fall, and because of that, diseases associated with high cholesterol—such as heart disease—are better controlled (Science Daily, 2019). It was also found that this diet can slow the progression of diabetes as well as reducing the deaths following breast cancer. As one is encouraged to eat more high-fiber dishes to prevent feeling hungry, insulin can be better controlled as glucose is being released into the blood slower.

Cons

The weight loss is not as high as what is seen in carbohydrate-limiting diets and likely this diet is better suited to maintaining a set weight if one is going to make use of it for a long-term diet (Rayzelman, 2017). With the cutting back of high-fat meats, there may also be a deficiency in various vitamin B supplements as well as the mineral zinc. Cutting out too much fat will go against the body's need to absorb fat-soluble vitamins. Even if supplements are taken, the body will not be able to absorb them if there isn't enough fat to do so. There is also a concern about the mental health risks of this diet. If one restricts all kinds of fats, the brain will suffer. The human brain cannot function without healthy fats.

According to Richard Fogoros (2021), there isn't much scientific evidence that states that a low-fat diet is significantly better than any other diet. This is not to say that it doesn't work for some people, but this is anecdotal evidence. If one wishes to make use of this diet, it is a very good idea to make sure that you are monitoring your calorie intake as well as continuing to consume healthy fats to maintain the body's health.

There is an argument that with lower cholesterol one's health will improve. However, according to Kris Gunners (2018a), the so-called bad cholesterol LDL's size is very important. The smaller the LDL molecule, the worse it is for your heart. He goes on to explain that a low-fat diet can change the LDL molecules from a large shape to a smaller one which causes more clogging in the arteries. Not only that, but the diet can reduce the HDL—the so-called good cholesterol—and increase the triglycerides in one's blood.

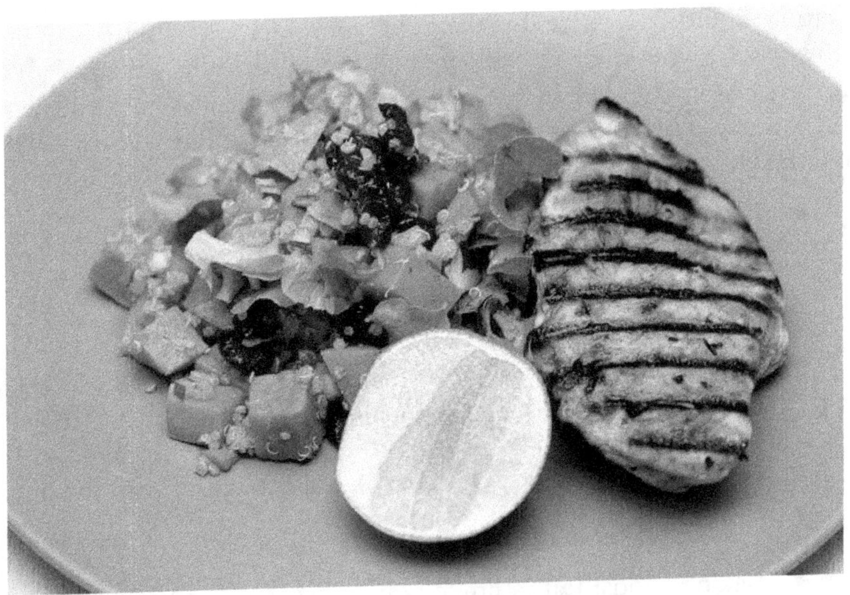

Duration

If you find that this diet works for you and you don't suffer any negatives, then you can remain on it for as long as you want. However, according to Kris Gunnars (2018a), the diet was never based on any scientific proof when the low-fat guidelines were first introduced to the American diet, and now with scientific experiments, there is even less evidence to support it.

This is likely not a diet that should be maintained for a long period but rather just long enough to lose the necessary weight before returning to a regular diet. Overall, it may just be a better idea to look at a person's whole diet and make healthier choices when it comes to your food habits. Seek a medical professional's advice on whether this is the diet for you before making use of it.

Shopping List

Cutting a little fat here or there in your diet has some benefits. However, if you want to follow this diet, under the guidance of a doctor, below you will find a list of products that will help you with this journey. This list was designed with the work of Rachel Nall (2019) and the website *Drugs.com* (2021):

- Fresh: No limit on any fruits and vegetables. Choose those higher in fiber to get the best benefits. If making use of canned options, then read the labels to ensure no hidden fats.

- Protein: Poultry (skin removed), fish, lean pork or beef, nuts, tofu (low-fat), seeds, and egg whites

- Dairy: All low-fat varieties, and make sure to limit consumption.

- Baking goods: Eat in limited quantities, and make sure they are made with low-fat products.

- Fats: Sunflower oil, peanut oil, canola oil, and olive oil; low-fat dressings

- Prepackaged goods: Avoid when possible or check labels.

- Grains: Whole grains, cereals (oats and barley), wild or brown rice

- Snacks: Popcorn, fruit, any low-fat options while monitoring the sugar levels

- Sauces and soups: Ensure they contain low-fat ingredients, or make use of homemade broths.

Vegetarians and vegans can also make use of this diet with the exclusion of animal products.

Meal Plan

Low-fat doesn't mean boring. There are many ways to get around not being able to make use of your favored cream sauces or toppings. A little bit of planning and creativity goes a long way with this diet. Remember that you cannot cut all fats out of your diet. Make use of the healthier oils to add a touch of fat to your salads or cooking. This way you can ensure that you can absorb all those fat-soluble vitamins that your body needs. To keep both your fat and cholesterol levels as low as possible the works of *Pritikin* (2016), Rachel Nall (2019), and Emily Lachtrupp (2020b) were used to design the following meal plan:

	Breakfast	Lunch	Dinner	Snacks
Day 1	Oatmeal with honey, fresh berries, and raisins, with a cup of orange juice.	Sweet potato with a touch of Dijon mustard with a salad made of lettuce, red onions, grilled tofu, and cherry tomatoes. Drizzle with Balsamic vinegar.	Skillet lemon chicken and potatoes with kale (one serving), if still hungry add a small green salad seasoned only with a pinch of salt and pepper.	¼ cup unsalted dry-roasted almonds and one medium pear.
Day 2	Cinnamon overnight oats (one	Slow-Cooker Mediterranean stew (one	Veggie burger patties topped roasted red	Carrot sticks with hummus

	serving) with one cup of nonfat plain Greek yogurt.	serving) and a large pear.	peppers on a bed of lettuce or spinach.	dip.
Day 3	A 3-ounce serving of tofu scrambled with seasoning of choice with ½ a whole grain bagel.	A whole wheat wrap with tuna (in brine), cucumber, and a boiled egg, with a ¼ cup low-fat plain Greek yogurt.	Stuffed sweet potato with hummus dressing (one serving).	Medium pear, apple, and a cup of grapes.
Day 4	Apple and peanut butter toast (one serving).	Cream of broccoli soup.	Whole grain spaghetti with tomato sauce, vegetables, and lean meatballs or vegetarian meatballs.	Passion fruit or pineapple and a handful of unsalted nuts of choice.
Day 5	Yogurt berry parfait.	Sweet Potato, kale, and chicken salad with peanut dressing (one serving) and one clementine.	Cauliflower shells with cheese.	A few whole grain or multi-seed crackers.
Day	A two-egg	Veggie and	Salmon with	Corn on the

| 6 | white omelet with freshly made salsa and chopped green onions. | hummus sandwich (one serving) and one medium orange. | sweet potato and broccoli (one serving). | cob and two slices of cantaloupe. |
| Day 7 | Grape and cashew salad sandwich. | ¾ cup edamame (soybean, whole), ¼ cup sliced celery, ¼ chopped cucumber, and a handful of diced radishes. If you want a dressing to go with that, make it with rice vinegar, a teaspoon of freshly grated ginger, and a pinch of wasabi. | Turkey and sweet potato chili and Guacamole chopped salad (one serving each). | Baby carrots and broccoli with Greek yogurt dip with seasonings such as salt, pepper, and lemon juice. |

If you find that you are still hungry during the day, then make use of fresh fruit and whole grain crackers for the added vitamins and fiber. For more low-fat recipes, look no further than *My Plate* which is filled to the brim with all kinds of recipes from breakfasts to even desserts and snacks. Each recipe shows not only the nutritional value of the meal but also the cost and the taste rating. Worth visiting if you want to start designing your own meals that are not only fat-free but delicious.

Chapter 6:

Zone Diet

What Is It?

This is another diet where one seeks to control the number of carbohydrates that are eaten per day. The macronutrients of the diet are consumed as 40% carbohydrates—concentrating on the low glycemic index (GI)—30% fats—concentrating on monounsaturated fats—and 30% proteins which should be lean. This diet was developed by Dr. Barry Sears as a way to reduce inflammation, lower the risk of chronic disease, slow down the aging process, lose weight fast, increase one's mental and physical performance (Raman 2017), as well as encouraging healthy insulin levels (Brazier, 2020b). This is considered a lifelong diet that encourages four main standpoints to be brought together to help a person get into the Zone lifestyle:

- Restrict calories but don't starve yourself: Restrict just enough calories to prevent the body from wanting to store the excess as fat. Avoiding overly processed foods will help with this pillar.

- Manage inflammation of the body: Inflammation is your immune system reacting, but if it reacts for too long, it becomes chronic inflammation which is bad for a person. Many people who follow this diet believe that some inflammation is good and even go as far as to take supplements to aid in it. This is one of the points that get tested—through a blood test—to show whether you are in the ideal zone for this diet or not.

- Make use of polyphenols: By eating a variety of fruits and vegetables—or making use of supplements that activates genes that are meant to enhance your well-being.

- Control gut microbes: These microbes are responsible for some of the inflammation in the body and can be managed through the use of fermentable fiber, omega-3, as well as polyphenol.

The diet has two ways you can follow it to get yourself into the Zone (Raman, 2017). The first is known as the hand-eye method—the beginner level—and then, for those that are a little more accustomed to the diet, the Zone food blocks. The hand-eye method is very simple to follow. You judge the food on your plate by roughly measuring it to your hand. An example of this would be:

- ⅓ of your plate should be a lean protein, roughly the size and thickness of your palm.

- ⅔ of the plate should be made up of low GI carbohydrates, avoiding starch vegetables where you can.

- A little fat should be added. Something like a drizzle of olive oil, a few almonds, or a slice or two of avocado.

Yvette Brazier (2020b) adds to this by saying there are some rules when it comes to the meals you prepare for yourself. These are:

- Within one hour of waking up, have a snack.

- Snacks and meals should be started with low-fat protein followed by foods that contain good fats and carbohydrates.

- The smaller and more frequent the meals the better. Upon eating the main meal aim to eat a snack within four hours, while if you eat a snack aim to eat a main meal within two hours, irrespective of whether you are hungry or not.

- Drink a minimum of eight glasses of water a day while eating plenty of omega-3 and polyphenol-rich foods.

If you are new to this diet, it is a good idea to start with the hand-eye method until you are more comfortable to move onto the Zone food block method which can be a little more complicated as there are measurements involved. If you feel comfortable trying this method, then you will need to measure your waist, hips, height, and weight, and put the information on *Dr. Sears' Zone Lab*: The Zone Body Fat Calculator. This site will calculate how many food blocks you will have available to you for the day.

On average, men will be allowed 14 blocks while women will be allowed 11, and these blocks make up the food you are allowed for the day. You can divide them up among the different meals you will have. Normally a snack will be one block while the main meal can vary from three to five blocks. Each block—protein, fat, and carbohydrate—has its quantity. Protein can be seven grams per block, fat is only 1.5 grams of an animal source or three grams of a plant source per block, while carbohydrates—measured as net carbs— can be nine grams per block. So, to remain with the correct ratio of protein to carbs to fats, you should have one block of protein, two blocks of carbs, and one block of fat.

The Zone food block method is considered the ideal way to get into the Zone that provides all the advantages of this diet. However, how does one know that they are in the Zone? There are a total of three tests that need to be done to achieve this:

- Triglycerides to HDL ratio: Simply put, comparing the bad cholesterol part to the good part. The lower the value, the better it is for your health. The Zone diet recommends a value less than one.

- Arachidonic acid (AA) to eicosapentaenoic acid (EPA) ratio: This is comparing one type of omega-6 to a type of omega-3. Omega-3 is considered to have anti-inflammatory effects so there should be more of it in your blood than omega-6. A ratio of between one and three is expected on this diet.

- HbA1c (glycated hemoglobin): This marker in your blood shows your average blood sugar level over the last three months, and you want this value to be fairly low. A value that is less than five percent is encouraged by the diet. The higher the marker the more likely it is that you are a candidate for diabetes.

Once all the numbers are where they need to be, then you are considered to be in the Zone and will get to enjoy the benefits of this diet.

Who Can Benefit?

The Zone diet actively encourages the consumption of fruits and vegetables while avoiding sugars and processed foods making this a diet, and albeit, a lifestyle, that many people can enjoy.

Pros

This diet is without extreme restrictions in terms of food which makes it an easy diet to plan meals around which are not only well-balanced but also include a variety of foods (Raman, 2017; Anderson, 2020). It is very similar to the Mediterranean diet though it does not encourage the consumption of grains of any kind. As long as the carbohydrates consumed are of the low GI variety, then any fruit and vegetables are allowed on the diet which makes for colorful plates that prevent people from becoming bored with eating the same old thing day in and day out.

The diet can be rather flexible depending on which of the two methods you prefer to make use of. If your aim is to lose weight rapidly, then sticking to the Zone food block method is a sure way to get rid of those pesky pounds that are packed around your waistline. This diet is also a sure way to control your blood glucose level by eating low GI foods which release sugars into the blood at a reduced rate (Brazier, 2020b).

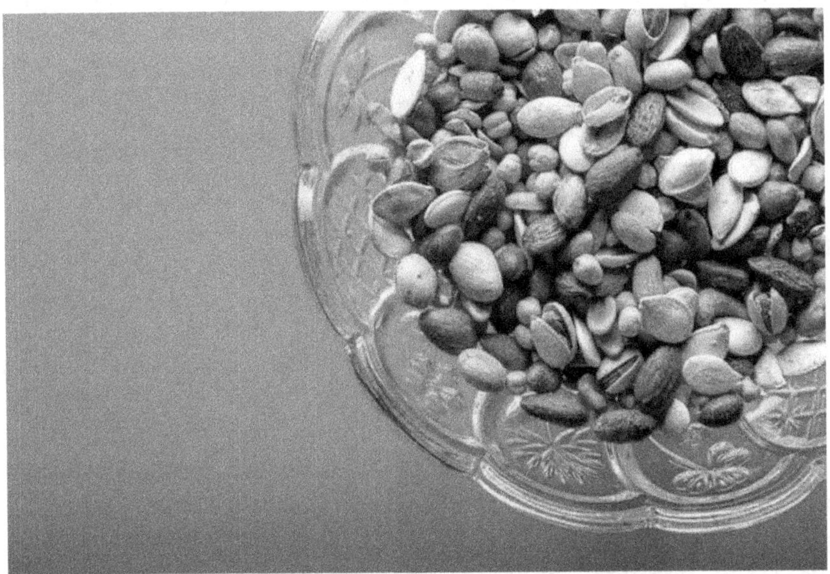

Cons

There is very little scientific evidence that proves what this diet claims it can do (Raman, 2017). Athletes who tried the diet stated that though they managed to lose weight, they found that their performance was lacking, and they often got tired before others who were not on the diet. There is also no scientific proof of significant inflammation reduction because of the diet, and Dr. Sears is not overly concerned about not lowering the amount of cholesterol that people eat on this diet (Brazier, 2020b).

Another worrying factor is that most suggestions for supplements for this diet are from products that are solely sold by the Zone brand (polyphenols and certain foods). The diet also does away with high-fiber grains, legumes, and certain fruits that can have an impact on the fiber content of the food, and thus can upset stomachs if not carefully monitored (Anderson, 2020).

Tracking of the macromolecules can also be fairly difficult as you need to be monitoring the grams of each to make sure that you remain in the Zone. This diet may not be for everyone who wants to benefit from the claims of warding off certain chronic diseases. If you are suffering from a chronic disease, speak to a physician before changing to a diet in hopes of a treatment.

Duration

This diet actively encourages making the right choices when it comes to your eating habits. Some people will treat it as a diet while for others it can become a lifestyle. With the guarantee of weight loss as well as a diminished waistline, this is the perfect diet for someone who wants to lose weight and keep it off. Once a person can keep track of what is needed in the diet, the worst part is perhaps finding good sources of low GI but high-fiber foods to help with any stomach issues that may occur. This may not be a diet for everyone, but it does have its merits and can become a good and healthy lifestyle for those that need a little more structure in their diet.

Shopping List

You will want to make use of a farmers' market to get access to a wide variety of fresh fruits and vegetables to help you with this diet. Make sure to check which of these are on the low GI scale before making any purchases. The list below is from suggestions of *WOD Fever* (n.d.), Ryan Raman (2017), and Yvette Brazier (2020b):

- Fresh: All fruits and vegetables should be low GI; the more colorful the better.

  - Vegetables: Bean sprouts, collard greens, okra, turnips, lentils, onion, tomatoes, lettuce, zucchini, etc. Avoid all starchy vegetables.

  - Fruits: Apples, kiwis, berries in general, all stone fruit—peaches, apricots, etc.—all citrus fruits, grapes, etc.

- Protein: Lean or low-fat protein is best, poultry breast without skin, lean beef, lean lamb, soy products, lean pork, egg whites, and seafood

- Dairy: Make use of low-fat varieties of milk, cheese, yogurt, and creams.

- Baking goods: Avoid completely if possible.

- Fats: Make use of monounsaturated fats, a variety of nuts, and kinds of butter made from them—peanuts, almonds, etc.—avocado, and canola oil.

- Prepackaged goods: Avoid all processed goods.

- Grains: Very limited amounts of barley and oatmeal

- Snacks: Stick to snacking on nuts and fruits.

- Sauces and soups: Homemade vegetable soups, nothing overly processed

The diet can accommodate those who are living a vegan or vegetarian lifestyle.

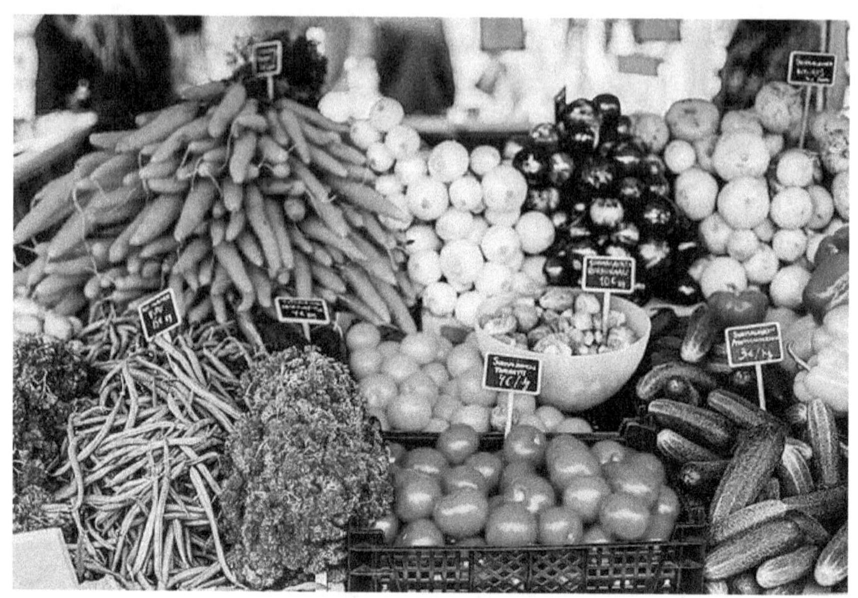

Meal Plans

The following meal plans take the guessing out of the Zone food blocks as each meal will be assigned a value to help you reach the number that you need to get for the day. However, if you are not comfortable with the food blocks, then refer back to the hand-eye method and create meals with the shopping list provided.

As a beginner, always try to make your plate colorful with a variety of vegetables and fruits, as these will provide you not only with your vitamins and minerals but also your polyphenols and fiber. If you find that you are not getting enough fiber in your diet, then look at making use of kale, spinach, or even cucumber to help regulate you. Play around with the food types to find which best suits your pocket, needs, as well as taste. The following meal plans—one for men totaling 14 blocks and one for women totaling 11 blocks, using similar foods—was designed using the work of "Meal Plan" (2004):

	Breakfast	Lunch	Dinner	Snacks
Day 1	Two corn tortillas with ½ cup black beans, ⅓ cup onions, chopped green pepper, three eggs (scrambled) two ounces of cheese, and five tablespoons avocado. (5 blocks)	Three ounces canned tuna (in brine) with three teaspoons light mayo and one slice whole wheat bread. Plus half a medium apple. (3 blocks)	Three ounces baked chicken breast with one and a half oranges and three macadamia nuts. (3 blocks)	¼ cup cottage cheese, ½ carrot, three celery stalks, and five olives. (1 block) One ounce chicken or tuna, one medium peach, and ½ tsp peanut butter. (1 block) A cup of strawberries, ¼ cup cottage cheese, and a macadamia nut. (1 block)
Day 2	Three-ounce steak, two eggs, with one slice of whole wheat bread with 1 ⅔ tsp butter, and	Two slices of whole wheat bread, 4 ½ ounces sliced deli meat, one ounce of cheese, and four tablespoons	Beef Stew: Fry together 1 ⅔ tsp olive oil, ¼ cup chopped onion, ½ green pepper,	¼ cup cottage cheese, ½ cup pineapple, and six peanuts. (1 block)

	1 ½ medium apples. (5 blocks)	avocado. (3 blocks)	and about 10 ounces beef. Then add a cup zucchini, a cup of mushrooms, and ½ cup tomato sauce Season with garlic, salt, and pepper, In addition to the main meal add two cups of fresh strawberries. (5 blocks)	
Day 3	¾ cup cottage cheese, ¼ cubed cantaloupe, a cup of strawberries, ½ cup of grapes, and a sprinkle of almond shavings. (3 blocks)	A corn tortilla, four ounces of cheese, four tablespoons guacamole, and sliced jalapeño then add salsa. Add one and half oranges to round the meal off. (4 blocks)	Sauté 7 ½ ounces fresh fish with 1 ⅓ cup zucchini in herbs. Serve with a large salad with 2 ½ tbsp salad dressing of choice and ¼ cup black beans on the side. Add two cups of fresh strawberries for dessert.	An ounce of sardines, ½ nectarine, and five olives. (1 block) Three ounces marinated and baked tofu, ½ a medium apple, and ½ teaspoon peanut butter. (1 block)

		(5 blocks)	
Day 4	A cup of cooked oatmeal, ½ cup grapes, ¾ cup cottage cheese, and two teaspoons walnuts. Add a tablespoon of protein powder with some vanilla and cinnamon for taste. (4 blocks)	4 ½ ounces of sliced deli meat, an ounce of cheese, one medium apple, one medium grapefruit, and four macadamia nuts. (4 blocks)	Five ounces of turkey breast and 2 ½ cups of kale. Sauté the mixture with 1 ⅔ tsp olive oil, garlic, and crushed red peppers. Add three medium peaches as dessert. (5 blocks)	One ounce hummus serving, ½ a tomato, and 1 ½ ounce serving of feta cheese. (1 block)
Day 5	½ pita bread with two scrambled eggs, two ounces of cheese, one ounce of ham, and one and a half apples. (5 blocks)	Two slices of bread, 4 ½ ounces of deli meat, two ounces of cheese, five tablespoons, and half a medium apple. (5 blocks)	Two-ounce baked chicken breast, 1 medium orange, and two macadamia nuts. (2 blocks)	A poached egg, ½ slice of whole wheat bread, and ½ tsp peanut butter (1 block) A hard-boiled egg and a large spinach salad with a teaspoon oil

			and vinegar dressing. (1 block)
Day 6	Blend two cups of milk, three tablespoons protein powder, two cups frozen strawberries, ½ cup frozen blueberries, and 20 almonds. (5 blocks)	Four ounces grilled chicken, two cups lettuce, ¼ tomato. ¼ cucumber, ¼ green pepper, ½ cup black beans, and ¼ cup kidney beans, all drizzled with two tablespoons salad dressing. (4 blocks)	Three-ounce roasted turkey breast with 2 ½ cups steamed kale. Cook with a teaspoon olive oil, garlic, and crushed red peppers. As dessert, add a peach. (3 blocks)	One-ounce grilled turkey breast, ½ cup blueberries, and three cashews (1 block) One-ounce piece of cheese, ½ a medium apple, and one macadamia nut. (1 block)
Day 7	½ pita bread, two fried eggs, an ounce of grated cheese, an ounce of ham, and one medium apple. (4 blocks)	Four ounces of tuna with four teaspoons of light mayonnaise on a slice of whole wheat bread and a medium apple. (4 blocks)	This recipe serves three people. Cook together ⅔ cup onion, two green peppers with garlic, cumin, chili powder, and crushed red peppers. Then add 18	A cup of strawberries, ¼ cup of cottage cheese, and a macadamia nut. (1 block) One ounce of jack cheese, a tablespoon of

			ounces of ground beef until browned. Next, add two cups of tomato sauce, a cup of black beans, a cup of kidney beans, and about 40 olives, destoned and cut up. Add fresh cilantro to taste. (4 blocks)	guacamole, and one tomato. (1 block)

This is an example of a 14 block Zone food block diet for men. The diet below is an 11 block meant for women using the same meals as what was described for the men:

	Breakfast	Lunch	Dinner	Snacks
Day 1	A corn tortilla, ¼ cup black beans, one scrambled egg, one ounce of cheese, and a tablespoon of avocado. (2 blocks)	Three ounces canned tuna (in brine) with three tsp light mayo and one slice whole wheat bread. Plus half a medium apple.	Cook together ⅔ cup onion, two green peppers with garlic, cumin, chili powder, and crushed red peppers. Then add 18 ounces of ground beef until browned. Next, add two	In a cup of water add a tbsp of spirulina, a cup of frozen berries, and three cashews. Blend everything. (1 block) ¼ cup cottage

		(3 blocks)	cups of tomato sauce, a cup of black beans, a cup of kidney beans, and about 40 olives, destoned and cut up. Add fresh cilantro to taste (serves three). (4 blocks)	cheese, a cup of strawberries, and a macadamia nut. (1 block)
Day 2	Grill a three-ounce steak and an egg Served on a slice of whole wheat with 1 ⅓ tsp butter added. On the side, have ½ a cantaloupe. (4 blocks)	Two slices of whole wheat bread, 4 ½ ounces sliced deli meat, one ounce of cheese, and four tablespoons avocado. (3 blocks)	Grill a 4 ½ ounce serving of fish while frying 1 ⅓ cup zucchini. Serve with a large salad drizzled with 1 ½ tablespoons of salad dressing. For dessert have a cup of fresh strawberries. (3 blocks)	¼ cup cottage cheese, ½ cup pineapple, and six peanuts. (1 block)
Day 3	¾ cup cottage cheese, ¼ cubed cantaloupe,	A corn tortilla, four ounces of cheese, four tablespoons	Cook ¼ cup of onion, ½ a chopped green pepper, four ounces cubed	An ounce of sardines, ½ nectarine, and five olives.

	a cup of strawberries, ½ cup of grapes, and a sprinkle of almond shavings. (3 blocks)	guacamole, and sliced jalapeño then add salsa. Add one and half oranges to round the meal off. (4 blocks)	beef, and ⅔ olive oil. Then add ½ cup of zucchini, a cup of mushrooms, and ¼ cup tomato sauce then allow to simmer. Season with garlic, salt, and pepper. (2 blocks)	(1 block) Three ounces marinated and baked tofu, ½ a medium apple, and ½ teaspoon peanut butter. (1 block)
Day 4	¾ cubed cantaloupe, ¾ cup cottage cheese, and nine almonds. (3 blocks)	4 ½ ounces of sliced deli meat, an ounce of cheese, one medium apple, one medium grapefruit, and four macadamia nuts. (4 blocks)	Grill a 4 ½ ounce fresh fish then sauté 1 ⅓ cup zucchini in herbs. Together serve with 1 large salad drizzled with 1 ½ tablespoons salad dressing. Follow up with a dessert of a cup of fresh strawberries. (3 blocks)	One ounce hummus serving, ½ a tomato, and 1 ½ ounce serving of feta cheese. (1 block)

Day 5	A cup of cooked oatmeal, ½ cup grapes, ¾ cup cottage cheese, and two tsp walnuts. Add a tablespoon of protein powder with some vanilla and cinnamon for taste. (4 blocks)	Four ounces grilled chicken, two cups lettuce, ¼ tomato. ¼ cucumber, ¼ green pepper, ½ cup black beans, and ¼ cup kidney beans, all drizzled with two tablespoons salad dressing. (4 blocks)	Bake a two-ounce chicken breast and serve with an orange and two macadamia nuts. (2 points)	A poached egg, ½ slice of whole wheat bread, and ½ tsp peanut butter. (1 block)
Day 6	½ pita bread, two fried eggs, an ounce of grated cheese, an ounce of ham, and one medium apple. (4 blocks)	Three ounces deli meat, one ounce of cheese, one and a half apples, and three macadamia nuts. (3 points)	Two-ounce baked chicken breast, 1 medium orange, and two macadamia nuts. (2 blocks)	One-ounce grilled turkey breast, ½ cup blueberries, and three cashews (1 block) One-ounce piece of cheese, ½ a medium apple, and one macadamia nut.

				(1 block)
Day 7	Blend a cup of milk with a tablespoon of protein powder, a cup of frozen strawberries, and 10 cashews. (2 points)	Four ounces of tuna with four teaspoons of low-fat mayonnaise on a slice of whole wheat bread and a medium apple. (4 blocks)	Three-ounce roasted turkey breast with 2 ½ cups steamed kale. Cook with a tsp olive oil, garlic, and crushed red peppers. As dessert, add a peach. (3 blocks)	A cup of strawberries, ¼ cup of cottage cheese, and a macadamia nut. (1 block) One ounce of jack cheese, a tablespoon of guacamole, and one tomato. (1 block)

If you are interested in learning more about the Zone diet, want access to more recipes, as well as the products that are promoted by Dr. Sears, then look no further than here.

Chapter 7

Dukan Diet

What Is It?

Unlike the other diets discussed so far, this is a high-protein, low-carb, and low-fat diet. This diet gets even more complicated in the fact that you can only consume about 100 different types of foods (Brazier, 2020c). Of those foods, 32 are vegetables—used in the second phase of the diet—while 68 are protein-based, which are used in the initial phase of the diet. There is no limit on how much you can eat of these foods, but they need to be these foods only. Additional foods not from the list can only be added during the later stages of the diet. Essentially, according to Ayren Jackson-Cannady (2013), the heart of this diet comes down to oat bran (very limited), lean protein, and a daily 20-minute walk. Walking is not only rewarding when it comes to the view, it also works off those excess calories so that you can enjoy your meals guilt-free.

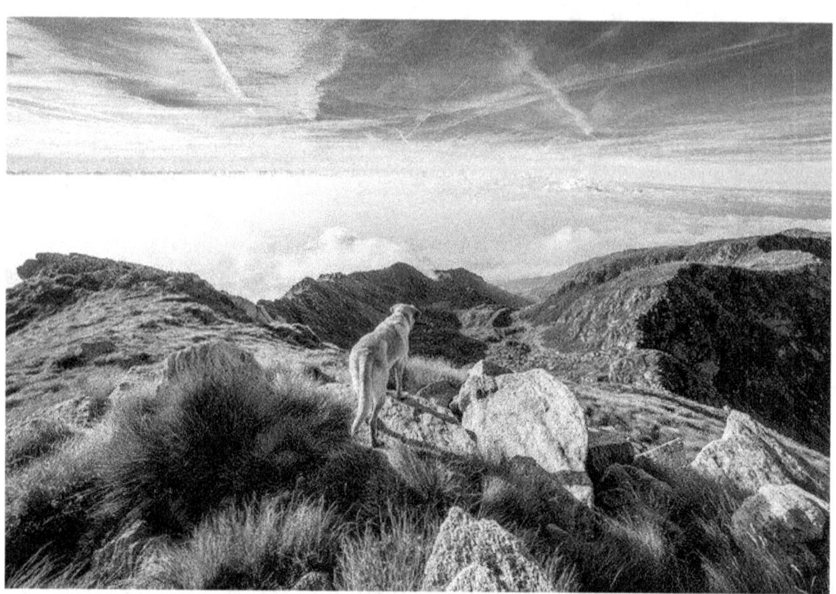

The Dukan diet is a little similar to the Atkins and keto diet as one is severely limiting the carbohydrate amounts that are eaten. However, because fats are also being restricted, the body is forced into a starvation-like mode where it is forced to use the stored fats as a form of energy. By making use of lean protein, people tend to lose weight because it is low in fat and thus has fewer calories. Digestion of protein requires more energy, so more calories are being burned. Also, protein makes a person feel fuller for longer so you do not feel hungry. Thus, you eat less because you feel full while taking in fewer calories and using more calories to burn through what you are eating. Not only is your food carefully monitored, but exercise is crucial to this diet which is something no other diet discussed so far has required as part of its process.

This diet has four phases that require specific things to be eaten to achieve weight loss (Spritzler, 2018; Brazier, 2020c; Dolson, 2021):

- Attack phase: This phase can last anywhere from two to five days but if you are looking to lose more than 40 pounds then the suggested duration is seven days. You can only consume lean protein—the 68 choices that are on the may eat list—

during this time. These proteins need to also be low fat to achieve this phase correctly. Eat until you are full as there is no calorie counting needed. Other things that are required on this diet are that one must eat 1.5 tablespoons of oat bran, for fiber requirement, drink 1.5 liters of water, and exercise for 20 minutes every day. In theory, one should be losing weight rapidly.

- Cruise phase: This phase is to support the gradual weight loss by adding the 23 types of vegetables that are allowed on this diet. One can decide to have pure protein days while alternating with protein and vegetable days. This part of the diet can be for several days up to several months depending on how much weight you want to lose. It is said that three days on the cruise phase will allow for one pound lost. As long as the vegetables are non-starchy, there is no limit on how much you can eat. There is also the addition of two tablespoons of oat bran and the exercise should now be for between 30 and 60 minutes a day, and keep drinking a total of 1.5 liters throughout the day.

- Consolidation phase: This phase is not about losing weight but keeping off what you have already lost thus far. Now, one may make use of starchy vegetables and even whole grain bread, which should remain at one to two portions only. This will remain limited while the 100 foods on the list can still be eaten with no limit. Another thing that sets this diet apart from those previously mentioned is that you may make use of up to two celebratory meals a week. This can consist of an appetizer, main dish, a dessert, and a glass of wine if one is so inclined (Spritzler, 2018). It is also suggested that one chooses a day out of the week—the day needs to be the same every week—to only eat from the attack phase protein list. There also needs to be the consumption of 2.5 tablespoons of oat bran, 1.5 liters of water, and about 25 minutes of exercise a day.

- Stabilization phase: This is your long-term plan where you shouldn't be picking up any excess weight but you also shouldn't be losing any. There still needs to be a pure protein day—make sure that it is the same day of the week every week—exercise for 20 minutes, have three tablespoons of oat bran, and keep drinking 1.5 liters of water every day. At this stage of the diet, it can become a lifestyle if one wishes so.

The oat bran is important for fiber, as pure protein has none, and the water is vital to prevent dehydration as the body uses the stored glycogen which in turn causes the loss of water. The use of exercise every day also helps to keep the metabolism high. This does not need to be high-intensity training, as a walk is suitable.

Who Can Benefit?

This diet is very strict on what you can and can't eat. If someone is not used to a highly restrictive diet or cannot make time to exercise daily, this is likely not the diet for you. Vegans and vegetarians will struggle with this diet, but it is possible. This is because foods such as nuts, lentils, and beans are not on the list of foods that are allowed (Jackson-Cannady, 2013). These people will have to make use of tempeh, tofu, or seitan which can lead to rather boring meals.

Pros

There are quite a few advantages when on the Dukan diet. Being on a high protein diet allows for rapid weight loss, an increase in calories burned because of gluconeogenesis, and an increase in the metabolic rate (Spritzler, 2018). Not only that, but protein makes one feel fuller for longer because the hunger hormone that triggers the need to eat—ghrelin—is suppressed. This diet also forces one to give up all processed foods during the first two phases while limiting them in the last two. As one is eating fewer carbohydrates, one is also improving the glucose balance in the blood which is a great way to deal with type 2 diabetes or prediabetes (Brazier, 2020c).

Daily exercise is encouraged on this diet (Jackson-Cannady, 2013) which in itself is something many people need encouragement in. If one is sensitive to gluten, this is a great diet for you as the first two stages of the diet are completely gluten-free. Shopping is also easier as there are only 100 different kinds of foods that you can buy to eat from.

The diet is also very predictable, as you decide how much weight you want to lose—true or ideal weight—and then remain on the first two phases of the diet for the amount of time required to lose the excess weight you have set out to lose. This diet also shies away from the use of salt which in turn will help with high blood pressure (Dolson, 2021).

Cons

There isn't much scientific research to match the claims that are made on this diet (Spritzler, 2018). This is a highly restrictive diet that is very low in fiber and generally makes for a boring diet if you are not creative with your food preparation (Jackson-Cannady, 2013). If you are a person who has gout, liver, or even kidney issues, this is not the diet for you, as the waste products of the diet will cause problems. There is also a chance of dehydration if you do not drink the volume of water that is prescribed on this diet (Brazier, 2020c). Some of the lean meats on the diet can become expensive to purchase, so it is a good idea to keep an eye out for specials and then freezing the excess.

The weight loss on Dukan can also be attributed to exercising daily and not just the foods that are consumed. Because of the restrictive nature of this diet, there may be issues with getting the correct balance of vitamins and nutrients needed by a person, so supplements may be necessary. Lastly, there should be next to no salt used on this diet which can cause food to not be as tasty as it would be with it (Dolson,

2021). This is also a fairly complicated diet that requires you to determine how long you need to be on the various phases.

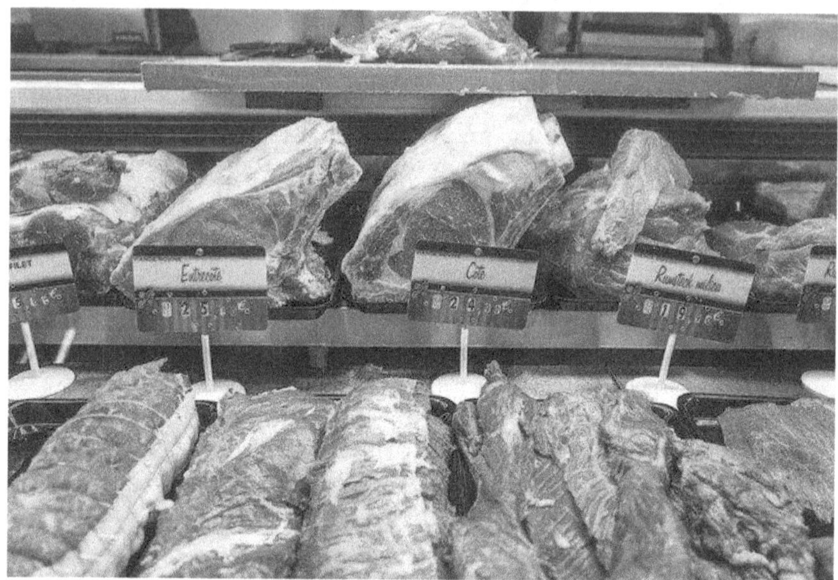

Duration

For people who do not have preexisting conditions for liver and kidneys, this is a diet that can help with a set amount of weight that needs to be lost. However, as this diet may become boring with the limited food allowed on it, it is not considered the type of diet that everyone could make a lifestyle out of.

Shopping List

The first thing that is very important to know is what you are allowed to eat. In the table below, provided by *Dukan Diet.com*, you will find the 68 different proteins and 32 vegetables—which you will only make use of in the Cruise phase—that you are allowed to eat for the first two phases of the diet.

Meat	Beef: Tenderloin, flank steak, sirloin, London broil, filet mignon, lean slices of roast beef, veal chops, veal scaloppine, and extra-lean Kosher beef hot dogs
	Pork: Reduced-fat bacon, extra-lean ham, lean center-cut pork chops, tenderloin, loin roast
	Venison: All meat cuts
	Buffalo: All meat cuts
	Poultry: Chicken liver, low-fat deli slices of chicken or turkey, ostrich steak, quail, wild duck, Cornish hen, turkey, fat-free turkey, and chicken sausages
	Fish: Arctic char, haddock, catfish, cod, flounder, grouper, herring, perch, fresh or smoked halibut, mackerel, monkfish, orange roughy, fresh or canned (in water) sardines and tuna, sea bass, sole, surimi, swordfish, tilapia, trout, shark, mahi-mahi, red snapper, and fresh or smoked salmon
	Shellfish: Squid, clams, crab,

	crawfish, lobster, crayfish, mussels, oysters, octopus, scallops, and shrimp
Vegan / Vegetarian-friendly protein	Seitan, soy-based foods, veggie burgers, tempeh, soy bacon, tofu
Dairy (all fat-free)	Cottage cheese, sour cream, cream cheese, milk, ricotta, and plain Greek-style yogurt
Eggs	Quail, duck, and chicken
Miscellaneous	Sugar-free gelatin (Jelly)
Vegetables (Cruise phase onward)	Artichoke, asparagus, bean sprouts, green beans, broccoli, brussels sprouts, cabbage, carrot, beet, cauliflower, celery, cucumber, eggplant, endive, fennel, kale, spinach, watercress, rhubarb, lettuce, arugula, radicchio, squash, mushrooms, okra, onions, tomato, leeks, shallots, palm hearts, peppers, pumpkin, radishes, spaghetti squash, turnip, and zucchini

For the Attack phase, make use of everything except for the vegetables, which should only be incorporated in the Cruise phase. The remaining items on your shopping list—for the remaining phases—should include some of the following (Spritzler, 2018):

- Fresh: Continue to make use of the vegetables in the table above. From the Consolidation phase, you can make use of one serving—approximately 3.5 ounces—a day of berries, pear, apple, kiwi, apricot, plum, peach, orange, melon, or nectarines.

- Protein: Continue with everything listed in the table above. There is an allowance of roast lamb up to twice a week.

- Dairy: A serving of cheese (1.5 ounces) a day is allowed.

- Starch: One to two servings (about eight ounces) a week of foods such as potatoes, beans, rice, other grains, and legumes

- Fats: Avoid all excess where possible.

- Grains and bread: Oat bran is a must for all of the phases of the diet, and try up to two slices of whole grain bread a day with reduced butter if wanted.

- Snacks: There should be no need for snacks; if you are hungry, increase the number of items you eat from the table.

- Eating out: Make use of your up to two celebratory meals a week if you want.

To avoid possible boredom on this diet, one should try to eat a variety of protein types and vegetables—on the Cruise phase—and not the same meal which is easily prepared. Boredom on a diet will cause one to give it up. Add very small amounts of oil (one teaspoon) and salt to the cooking process. Artificial sweeteners are allowed if needed for coffee and tea.

Meal Plan

Below will be a meal plan for the first four days on the Attack phase and then three days on the Cruise phase. If you need more time on the

Attack phase, simply add your protein-packed meals until you reach seven days. Not all vegetables need to be cooked, so if you are missing the crunch of your favorite snacks, try eating some raw veggies with your protein. Remember to eat till you are full, irrespective of the phase you are in. Follow the rules for each of the phases—drinking water, consuming the oat bran, and exercising—and you will succeed. The following meal plan, and recipes, were put together with the works of *My Dukan Diet* (n.d.-b) and Louise Atkinson (2011):

	Breakfast	Lunch	Dinner	Snacks
Day 1	Low-fat cottage cheese with two slices of grilled chicken breast.	400 g Vietnamese beef with some low-fat yogurt.	Four hard-boiled eggs served with Dukan mayonnaise.	Pink cheesecake cupcakes.
Day 2	Three-egg omelet with several slices of ham (less than five percent fat).	A grilled chicken breast with a side of muesli ice cream.	Garlic tiger prawns and chicken slices.	Cheese and ham roll-ups.
Day 3	Low fat yogurt with oat bran.	Grilled turkey breast steaks with ham slices.	Roast chicken (without skin).	Surimi sticks (fish or meat paste).
Day 4	Mint and curry omelet.	Steamed fish with herbs with a side of low-fat	Peppered beef steak	Oat bran cookies.

		cottage cheese.		
Day 5	Scrambled eggs with smoked salmon.	Take 175 g of extra-lean ham and spread 2 cups of fat-free cottage cheese over the slices. Then chop some chives, marjoram, and four shallots, finely, and sprinkle over. Roll the ham up and add Tabasco to taste. (serves 4)	Bake 800 g white fish fillets until cooked then add to a blender with 2 ½ cups fat-free fromage frais (fresh curd cheese), four eggs, five tbsp chopped herbs. Remove mixture and bake until eggs are fully cooked. (serves 4)	Cinnamon oat bran pancake.
Day 6	Oat bran porridge with skim milk and sweetener if desired.	750 g minced beef, an onion, two garlic cloves, a tbsp Worcestershire sauce, two tablespoons rosemary, 1–2 tablespoons mint (herbs	Steak and vegetables.	A serving of favored fruit.

		finely chopped), and one lightly beaten egg. Mix all ingredients and cook patties to the consistency wanted. Serve with a green salad (optional). (serves 3)		
Day 7	Whole wheat toast with two poached eggs.	Grilled chicken with a mixed vegetable salad.	Take 800 g chicken breasts and cut them into kebab-sized chunks. Then take an onion, one garlic clove, one tablespoon ginger, two tablespoons lemon juice, ½ tablespoon ground coriander, ½ tablespoon ground cumin, a teaspoon garam masala, two tablespoons	Oat bran muffins.

			coriander, and ½ cup fat-free plain yogurt and blend until smooth. Mix the chicken with marinade and refrigerate for two hours for threading the chicken onto the skewers and grilling until cooked. (serves 4)	

If bran oat is used in a recipe for the day, do not take in extra oat bran as it will affect the Attack phase of this diet. If hungry, eat as much as you want from the table of 100 items you are allowed to eat from and not just from the shopping list when in the Consolidation phase.

Chapter 8

Raw Food Diet

What Is It?

This diet is very similar to the raw food vegan diet where one is encouraged to eat all types of fruit, vegetables, nuts, and seeds raw (Jones, 2017). The food eaten is only considered raw if it has never been subjected to heat over 104–118 °F. The food should also be unpasteurized, not refined in any manner, or treated with pesticides. To prevent the diet from being too boring, the food can be prepared in several ways such as blending, juicing, drying, soaking, or even allowing for sprouting—for grains and some beans (Brazier, 2020d). The reason this diet is so popular is that many people believe that when you cook food, the nutrients and enzymes that promote good health are destroyed and can even make food toxic (Robinson, 2013).

It is believed that by consuming all manner of raw foods that headaches and allergies will clear up, there will be an improvement in people who suffer from arthritis and diabetes, plus one will get a boost to the memory and immunity. Promoters of this diet even go as far as to say that supplements are not needed on this diet, as the raw food will give you everything that you will need to live a healthy life.

Although the diet is primarily a vegan-like diet, vegetarians can make use of the diet by consuming raw eggs and unprocessed dairy, while omnivores can make use of raw or dried meat. If you are someone that is trying to avoid processed foods, this is a diet that may help you do that.

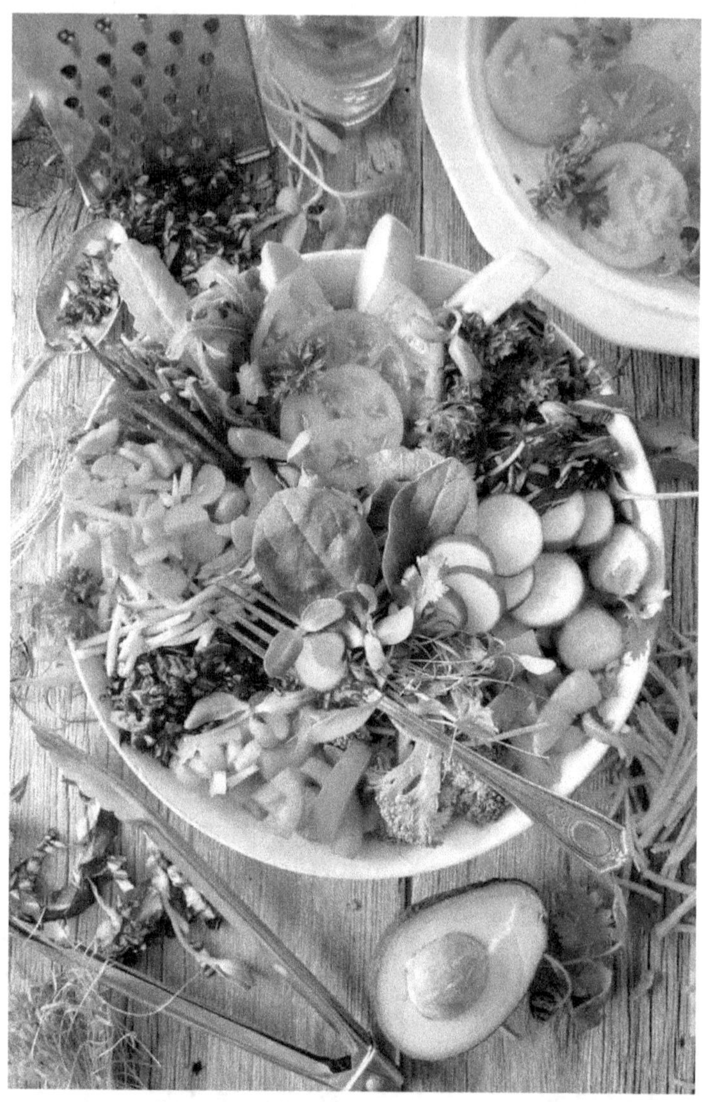

Who Can Benefit?

Many people can benefit from this diet to improve their fiber intake as well as vitamins and minerals that are readily available in fruits and vegetables. However, some foods are simply not safe to be eaten raw or unpasteurized.

Pros

A diet that makes use of raw fruits and vegetables ensures that water-soluble vitamins are consumed in abundance without them being destroyed in the cooking process. Fresh fruits, vegetables, nuts, and legumes all provide vitamins, minerals, proteins, healthy fats, and carbohydrates. There are no processed fats, salts, or sugars in this diet which means there will be less inflammation in the body. With the high level of fiber in the raw food diet, one will feel fuller for longer, plus raw foods generally contain fewer calories than those that have been cooked with other foods like oil. There is a claim by the followers of this diet that the enzymes present in the raw food are preserved when not cooking and thus a person can benefit from them. However, these enzymes are not only heat intolerant but also pH intolerant, so when the food hits the stomach acid, the enzymes are denatured anyway. Other advantages of this diet include better digestion, clear skin, as well as a person having far more energy (Brazier, 2020d).

By being on this diet, you will no longer be able to eat food that is considered "junk" by many, such as high-sugar content—soda and candy—or high-fat content food. There is also a large amount of body fat reduction on this diet due to the low-calorie intake (Jones, 2017).

The health benefits in fighting chronic ailments are also noted by Kara Mayer Robinson (2013). This diet is naturally low in sodium—found in many processed foods—and thus helping with lowering blood pressure as well as chances of stroke, heart problems, heart and kidney diseases. The loss of weight also helps with managing type 2 diabetes.

Cons

One of the main things that people believe about this diet is that cooking food makes it toxic. There is no scientific research that backs this claim at all. In fact, there are several foods that should be cooked, as eating them raw can lead to problems i.e., buckwheat, kidney beans, and even cassava (Brazier, 2020d). Not only that but bacteria like *Salmonella*, *Listeria*, and *E. coli* can cause severe foodborne diseases which cause food poisoning. Because of this, the diet is not suggested for anyone who has a compromised immune system, the very young and old, as well as anyone who may be pregnant (Robinson, 2013).

The preparation for the food can also take some time, especially if one is making use of drying or sprouting certain food types. Kitchen hygiene is a must if you are preparing raw foods to prevent the possible spread of bacteria from one source to another. All fruits and vegetables *must* be washed before consumption.

Although this diet does cause a drop in weight and cholesterol, this isn't always good. The overall drop in cholesterol that is noted is for all the cholesterol types, including HDL (Jones 2017). Severe weight loss, which has been noted on this diet, can cause a variety of issues such as a loss in bone mass due to low calorie and protein intake, as well as irregular or even halting menstrual cycles (amenorrhea).

When one is eating a raw food diet, there are several nutritional deficits of which protein, calcium, vitamin B12 and D, iron, and omega-3 are the most well-known. There have even been cases of tooth erosion with people who are on this diet for a long period. This could be due to the tough nature of the foods that one has to chew. When food is cooked, it is softer and more digestible. Some foods even give more nutrients when cooked as seen with beta-carotene and lycopene (Robinson, 2013).

Lastly, getting enough calories to support an active body can be challenging on a raw food diet, as with the high amount of fiber, one feels full even though the caloric requirements are not reached.

Duration

Although this diet has several merits and is perfect as a short-term diet, it is suggested to not make it a lifestyle. Unless you are willing to put the work into preparing nutritionally balanced food—as well as maintaining the highest level of hygiene—this may be a very difficult long-term diet. Especially when many believers in this diet believe that one shouldn't make use of supplements to make up for the lack of nutrients in the diet. If you feel you need supplements, then make use of them.

Even though a lifestyle change to match this diet isn't easily accomplished having several raw food meals a week will be beneficial to anyone who needs to give up processed foods as well as getting more fiber and vitamins into their diet. This is also a very difficult diet to maintain if you like to eat out as you will need to check even salads to make sure nothing processed has been added to them. It is better to maintain this diet if you only eat from home.

Shopping List

Shopping for this diet can be rather easy unless you are trying to go organic as well as raw food. Looking for organic foods can pose a time-consuming search on your part as well as being rather expensive, but it is possible if this is the route you want to go. Your best option is to go to farmers' markets to get what you need, but keep in mind that all food needs to be washed to prevent bacteria from being brought into your kitchen. The following shopping list was put together with the works of *Berry Abundant Life* (n.d.), Cherie Soria and Dan Laderman (n.d.), and Taylor Jones (2017) but don't be afraid to add any of your favorites to the list:

- Fruits and vegetables: There is no limit on the fruits and vegetables that you can eat on this diet. As long as it can be consumed raw, then you can eat it. Be careful of some vegetables which can cause upset stomachs if eaten in large quantities i.e., broccoli. Even fermented vegetables like kimchi are allowed on the diet. Consider getting dried fruit if you are craving sweetness in your diet i.e., dates.

- Protein: Nuts and seeds, raw red meat—which can also be air-dried—raw fish like tuna and salmon. Do not eat raw chicken!

- Sprouting: Make use of sprouting legumes such as peas, chickpeas, lentils, and beans, as well as grains such as quinoa, buckwheat, and millet.

- Dairy and eggs: Only unpasteurized milk and eggs, consumed raw; making use of raw yogurt—made from unpasteurized milk— is also an option.

- Fats: Cold-pressed oils like olive oil or coconut oil

This diet is perfect for vegans but might be a little more difficult for vegetarians and omnivores. The basic rule of thumb for this diet is if it is processed or cooked, you can't eat it.

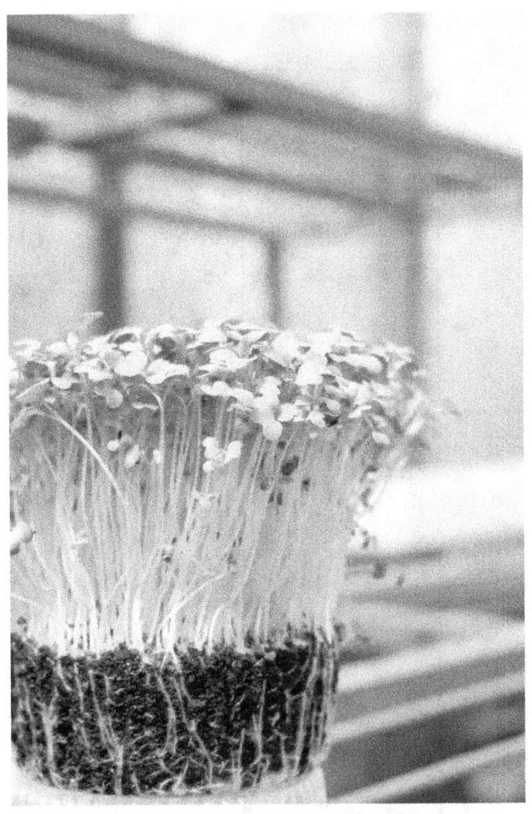

Meal Plan

There isn't much planning in making a meal but rather in planning to have the ingredients in your home before starting. You are spoiled for choice when it comes to the colors and tastes of your raw food. Look at adding some fresh herbs to your smoothies and dishes. Don't be afraid to experiment when it comes to getting the best out of the fresh diet. The following meal plan was created with the works of *One Green Planet* (n.d.), Alina Petre (2018), and Moira Lawler (2019):

	Breakfast	Lunch	Dinner	Snacks
Day 1	A tropical green spirulina smoothie.	Raw nori (seaweed) wraps with a spicy dipping sauce.	Raw lasagna with marinated vegetables, sun-dried tomatoes and a cashew-cilantro sauce.	Chia pudding and No-bake chocolate chip cookies.
Day 2	Two date energy balls with a serving of berries of choice.	Raw zucchini noodles with creamy garlic cashew sauce.	Raw vegan pizza	Trail mix with dried fruit and raw nuts.
Day 3	Breakfast smoothie and a portion of Chia seed pudding.	Rainbow salad (serves 4)	Lettuce or spinach wraps with patties made from raw sprouted lentil, topped with sprouted quinoa, diced peppers (all colors), tomatoes, cucumbers, and avocado.	Vegetable salad with a guacamole dressing.
Day 4	A large banana with two spoonfuls	Creamy butternut squash with marinated	Kale salad with diced vegetables, raw sprouted lentil	Triple berry cheesecake.

	of raw cashew butter.	mushrooms soup	patties, and cashew dressing.	
Day 5	Raw overnight oats with a spoonful of raw nut butter, banana slices, and berries of choice.	Kale salad served with fresh figs and oranges.	Raw Pad Thai.	Fruit of choice smoothies, raw milk, or raw yogurt can be used.
Day 6	Blackberry chocolate cake. (Yes! Cake for breakfast!)	Salad topped with broccoli, sliced carrots, and sprouts of choice.	Zucchini strips with fresh tomatoes, basil, and creamy cashew dressing.	A spoonful of raw almond butter with raw seeds, and a bowl of fruits of choice.
Day 7	Acai bowl with fresh fruit, nuts, seeds, and raw almond butter.	Greek salad with tomato, onion, cucumber, sprouted quinoa, olives, and cold-pressed olive oil.	Enchiladas with salsa, cheesy cashew sauce, and spicy nutmeat	Smoothie with banana, raw vegan protein powder, coconut water, and nut butter of choice.

Never let a meal plan limit you, as these are just suggestions. If you have favored foods, then by all means make use of them. Chop and change as you see fit on this diet, but keep an eye on your nutrients and supplement–if you wish–when necessary. If you are going to be making your own nut milk or butter, it is suggested that you purchase a good quality processor to help you.

Chapter 9:

Juice Diet

What Is It?

Out of all the diets, this is likely the easiest to follow and understand yet also one of the most restrictive. The juice diet, otherwise known as the juice cleanse, is a diet where all you practically need is a food processor or juicer and whatever fruits and vegetables you may want. Some people even opt to add supplements to their juice blends to make them healthier (Frey, 2020b). It is important to understand the difference between blending and juicing. Juicing is the liquid part that is produced from squeezing the fresh products together as well as removing all of the pulp—the fibrous floating parts—(Nall, 2018). A blend is where the pulp remains in the liquid. According to Cathy Wong (2021), many people who are staunch believers in this diet believe that antioxidants, phytochemicals, and even nutrients are more readily absorbed by the body if consumed in a liquid form.

Some juice diets can last from a single day up to 10 days (McCallum, 2020), and some of these diets even allow for smoothies or vegan snacks to add protein, fat, as well as other nutrients to be added (Wong, 2021). If you are new to the idea of a juice diet, it is not a bad idea to consider some snacks or raw food options to help you meet your nutritional needs. All the juice diets are considered "cleansing" and have the ability to detox your body. Even with that said, not one program makes mention of what toxins are being washed from your body on this diet nor is there any scientific backing for it. That is not to say it doesn't help people feel better for doing them, as it has already been established that a diet rich in fruits and vegetables does aid the body significantly in terms of minerals and vitamins. Not only that but when on a detoxing cleanse you are avoiding foods that are highly processed, contain refined sugar, and even caffeine.

A juice diet is more than just throwing random fruits and vegetables into a juicer and drinking whatever comes from it. It takes time and preparation before the cleanse, as well as having a change in diet after it to help with the maintenance of the cleanse (Project Juice, n.d.; Pasquale, 2013; Wong, 2021). There are a total of three stages:

- Preparation or Pre-cleanse stage: Take three to five days slowly removing certain foods from your diet and life. Avoid smoking (nicotine) while not consuming alcohol, any animal products (meat and dairy), caffeine, and all refined sugar. To compensate for the removal of these items, aim to add more water, fresh fruit, and vegetables. If you want to try more organic foods, you can do this, too.

- The Cleanse stage: This is the true start of the juicing diet and can last anywhere from one to three days, or longer if you deem it necessary. You need to be consuming a minimum of 32 ounces of juice, while some people say six to eight glasses of juice every 2-2 ½ hours while eating no solids at all. However, this can cause hunger pangs in some people that are too severe to control, so make sure you have some vegetables, fruits, or even soaked nuts to help you through this. Do not starve yourself, and take it slow or end the juice cleanse early if it is too difficult. Light exercise is encouraged to help with the diet.

- After the Cleanse: The day after you finish your cleanse, return to the diet you used before starting the cleanse. Within a day or two, you can start to add small portions of rice or even yogurt. After about five days, you can start to add in your lean meats, either red or white, back into your diet. As long as a person isn't pushing themselves too hard, exercise is also good during this time.

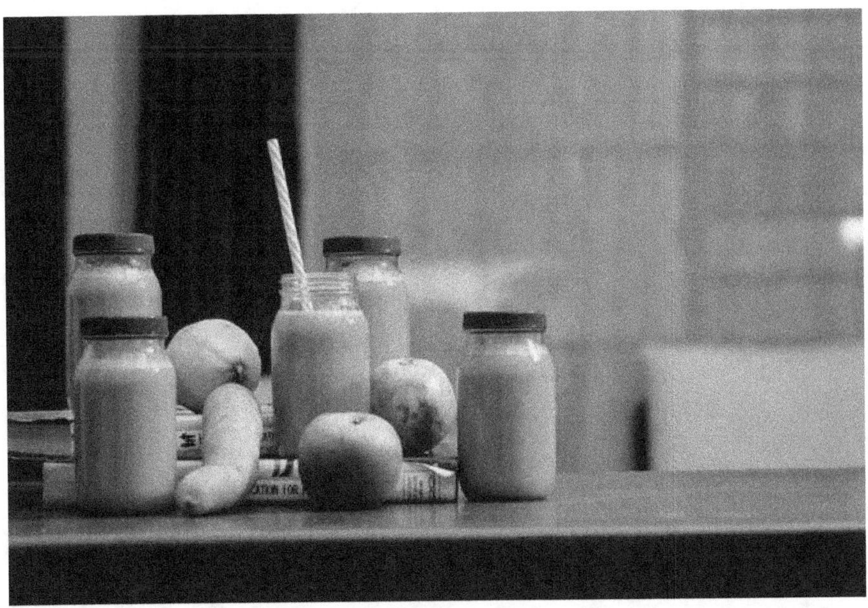

Just after the cleanse stage is a great opportunity to identify possible food allergies that may not have been previously identifiable without having to cut out different foods any way (Project Juice, n.d.). So if you are trying to establish a possible food allergy, ask your doctor if a juice diet is something that can help. You are not only encouraged to make use of a liquid diet but also to get a massage and practice body and mind wellness to help you with completing this diet. Many people who deal in traditional healing also state that one should be prepared for emotions that are associated with the organs such as the liver (anger), kidneys (fear), and gallbladder (frustration) which will be purged by the juice cleanse (Wong, 2021).

Who Can Benefit?

Many people can benefit from this diet, despite having no scientific evidence to back it. There is much anecdotal evidence that shows that this diet can be beneficial if controlled for a certain duration and a person doesn't force themselves into starvation or lacking too many nutrients and getting sick.

Pros

Consuming more fruits and vegetables has an improvement on one's health by allowing for better digestion due to the enzymes in the food (Frey 2020b; Wong, 2021). There is also the initial weight loss from switching to a liquid diet as well as giving the same benefits as fasting. Many believers say that the diet acts as detoxifying the body and that the toxins are flushed from your system but there is no current scientific proof of this. However, you will not be putting processed food, refined sugar, or caffeine in your diet, so that is a great benefit.

You will be consuming fewer calories which boosts weight loss and may even help with the motivation to lose more by choosing healthier options when it comes to food. The juices that are made are high in vitamins and minerals as well as anti-inflammatory compounds (Nall, 2018). These compounds help to boost the immune system to fight off diseases.

Cons

Any weight loss is temporary and will likely be regained once solid foods are consumed once more (Wong, 2021). The juice diets are generally very high in sugar (Frey, 2020b) in the form of fructose and can have an effect on the blood sugar if it is not maintained correctly (Wong, 2021). Even though the calories per glass consumed can be rather high (upward of 400 calories), it is hardly satisfying to drink every single meal. This dissatisfaction can lead to binge eating once the cleanse is completed (Frey, 2020b). Little to no fiber is being consumed so many cleanses have a laxative effect (Nall, 2018). This will lead to further nutrients lost as well as dehydration if a person is not careful.

Making one's own juice cleanses, or even some that are purchased, may have bacteria that cause foodborne diseases due to not being pasteurized. Because of this, the diet is not suggested for those that are very young or very old. The kidneys are also at risk as some vegetables are high in oxalates (Nall, 2018) which can cause kidney stones and damage the organs. Overall, one does not consume a lot of calories on this diet, and because of this, they can expect to feel headaches, hunger pangs, and a lot of fatigue.

This diet is severely limiting and because of that many nutrients are lacking. Some of these are vitamin B12, protein, and fats. Although, with the addition of fruit like bananas and avocados, this can be avoided. However, these are not fruits that can easily be juiced but rather would need to be blended and used in smoothies. Due to the lack of nutrients, there may be bone and muscle loss if one remains on this diet for too long (McCallum, 2020).

Duration

There is no denying that the juice diet has its place as a useful diet in terms of cutting out processed foods in favor of more fruits and vegetables but it is not a diet that can become a lifestyle. There is too much risk for organs like the kidneys if one remains on this diet for an extended period. However, the lower amount of calories consumed does teach a person to monitor their food intake. With the addition of finding possible food allergies, this diet is very useful if used for a short period. The duration isn't the only thing that is important for this diet but also the nutrients one requires to have a healthy, functional body.

If one carefully selects the fruits, vegetables, nuts, and maybe a few supplements here and there, this diet is perfect to break away from cravings and give your gut the rest it needs by reintroducing enzymes to help with its digestion after the cleanse is complete. A combination of a few days of juices, smoothies, and a few raw food snacks is likely the best way to get through this diet without suffering many of the disadvantages while enjoying the advantages.

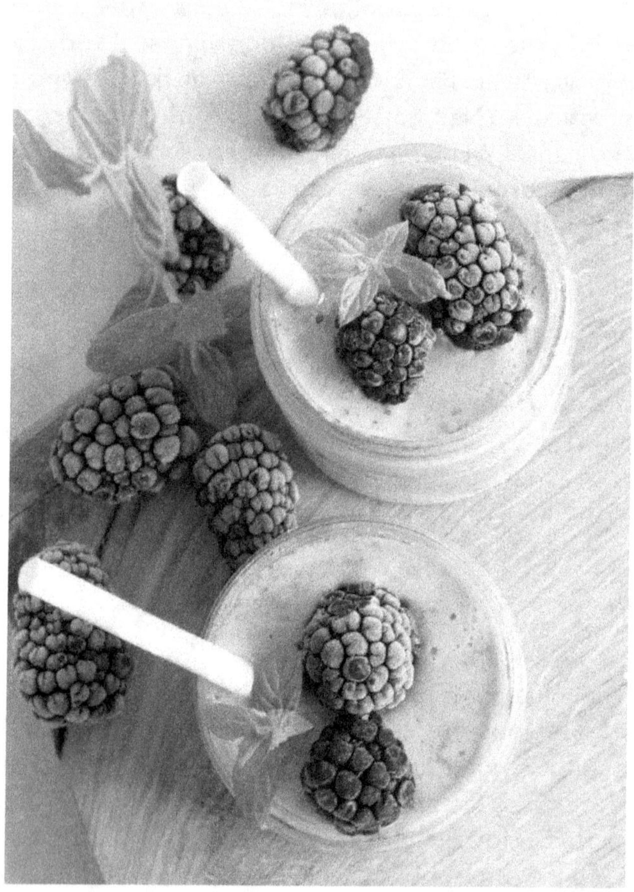

Shopping List

Many believers in the diet only call for organic fruits and vegetables, but this isn't necessary as it can get quite expensive. Make use of many fruits and vegetables that you find appealing and look at all possible combinations in terms of nutrients and taste to make the most out of this diet. If you find it necessary, especially if you aim for the longer cleansing part of the diet, do make use of vegetable broths, fresh snacks, or smoothies to help you get through it. Remember, this is about a better you, not unhappy and feeling sick all the time. One of your biggest purchases will be getting a food processor or juicer. Once you have the list of ingredients you need to buy, it is fairly simple. The below shopping list was designed with the works of Lacy Young (2012), *A Good Hue* (2013), and Nichole (2015) who used most of the ingredients in their own juice cleanse recipes:

- Fruit: All fruit can be used on this diet. If you are aiming for juicing only, then make use of fruits such as apples, pears, stone fruit, citrus, etc. If you are aiming for more smoothies, then make use of avocado and bananas. Dried fruits, such as dates, help give a sweet taste to any of the drinks you will make.

- Vegetables: Dark green leafy vegetables are a must but be careful of too many oxalates which can cause kidney stones. Any vegetable that can be eaten raw can be juiced, so avoid things like potatoes and corn. Even consider some sprouts to help with the protein levels.

- Nuts: These are great for smoothies but make sure that they have been soaked in water for about an hour or two before putting them through your juicer or food processor. Cashews and almonds are great for fiber and other nutrients. Different milk can also be added to smoothies if you need nce or nutrients.

- Herbs and spices: Cinnamon, turmeric, parsley, ginger, cayenne pepper, fennel, cilantro, cardamom, and nutmeg are all purely for taste, so you can make use of powdered or fresh forms.

- Miscellaneous: You can also use honey if you want.

Although there are many juice recipes online that you can make use of, don't be afraid to use your own imagination to come up with your own combinations. Some recipes can be stored for a few days, but it is strongly suggested that each juice is made freshly to prevent it from going bad. All fruits and vegetables need to be thoroughly washed to prevent contaminants from entering the healthy juices. Wash everything and when it doubt, peel skins.

If you only have a blender and not a juicer and you want to make use of the juices and not blends, then use a strainer or cheesecloth to remove most of the solids from the drink.

Meal Plans

The average juicing cleanse is about three days for most beginners, but one should prepare their diets before starting the juice diet. The meal plan below includes a three-day pre-cleanse followed by three days of the juice diet, then the final day where one is reintroducing foods to the diet. If you wish to follow a longer cleanse, then add one day extra onto the cleanse and see how you feel. If you feel that it is too difficult then remove one day from the cleanse. The pre-cleanse meal plan was designed with the works from *The Chalkboard* (2014) and *Clean Program* (n.d.):

	Breakfast	Lunch	Dinner	Snacks
Day 1	Carrot and tempeh sandwich.	Pistachio and persimmon salad.	A large Greek salad with extra olives and a drizzle of olive oil.	Fruits and nuts of choice.
Day 2	Mint chip smoothie and an apple.	Lentil burger with a large green salad with onions, tomatoes, and peppers.	Vegan summer rolls with a side place of preferred vegetables.	Roasted mixed nuts.
Day 3	Vegan breakfast hash.	Roasted stuffed apples with vegetables and pumpkin seeds.	Beet and lentil bowl.	Make a smoothie of your favorite fresh or frozen fruit.

The emphasis of the pre-cleanse is to make less and less use of animal products, processed foods, as well as addictive additives such as sugar and salt. This is also an opportunity for one to try to give up addictive behaviors such as drinking alcohol and smoking.

A total of five juices a day were chosen for this meal plan, but you can add one to two more a day if you are struggling to feel full. Otherwise, make use of some green tea upon waking and before going to bed. Cathy Wong (2021) suggests that the juices should be drunk at approximately 8 a.m. and 10:30 a.m. and in the afternoon at about 1 p.m., 3 p.m., 5 p.m., and 7 p.m. Although the meal plan below is of juices, you can make use of smoothies if you feel you are too hungry. Even include fruit, vegetables, nuts, or a pre-cleanse meal if the hunger is too much. Ensure that all the vegetables are washed and peeled before use. Fruit does not have to be peeled but has to be washed and cored if they contain seeds. This juice meal plan was created by Michelle Konstantinovsky (2014), Doug Hay (2021), and Breana Killeen (2021):

	Juice 1	Juice 2	Juice 3	Juice 4	Juice 5
Day 4	A large beet, 1-inch piece of ginger (peeled), a cup of tightly packed fresh spinach, 1 medium apple, and a medium carrot.	Three cups spinach, ½ cup fresh parsley, ½ a lemon (peeled), two medium pears, and six large celery stalks.	A beet, ½ cucumber, and dash of lime for taste.	5–6 large leaves of kale, 2–3 stalks of celery, ½ medium cucumber, a small lemon (peeled), and a small pear.	A cup chopped hearts of romaine lettuce, ¼ cup chives (chopped), two large tomatoes, ¼ fresh jalapeño (remove seeds), a large red bell pepper, two celery stalks, a medium carrot, and a cube of ice.
Day 5	A cucumber, three celery stalks, a	Five large carrots, two apples, a four-inch	Six fresh strawberries, a large cucumber, a large	A cantaloupe (peeled), three carrots, and	A large bunch of parsley, a large bunch of

	green apple, a green pear, three kale leaves, an orange (peeled).	piece of ginger (add more for taste if needed).	red apple, two medium carrots.	an inch of ginger root (peeled).	mint, a whole cucumber, and ½ medium green apple.
Day 6	¼–½ medium red cabbage, ½ small beet, a medium cucumber, and a red apple.	¼ medium red cabbage, a large cucumber, a cup of fresh blueberries, and a large red apple.	Two medium fennel bulbs, two green apples, a large handful of mint leaves, and a lemon (peeled).	1 ½ cups spinach, ½ grapefruit (peeled and pith—the white part—removed), two green apples, a 1-inch piece of fresh ginger (peeled), and two large stalks of celery.	Two celery stalks, a cucumber, and a medium tomato.

If you are making use of a lot of beets, do not be alarmed if you find that your urine has changed to pink. There is nothing to be alarmed about. However, if this continues after the juice cleanse and no more beets are being eaten, see a doctor immediately.

Now that your cleanse is completed, you can start to add more foods back into your diet. You can continue with the pre-cleanse meals, or you can start adding dairy and grains back into your diet. After a few days of this, you should be able to add lean meats to your diet once more.

	Breakfast	Lunch	Dinner	Snacks
Day 7	Muesli, low-fat yogurt, topped with berries or fruit of choice.	A small bowl of white rice with steamed vegetables of choice.	Berry blaster smoothie	Stick to fruit and vegetables for the first day after the juice cleanse.

Experiment with different fruits, vegetables, as well as herbs, and spices to make your own unique combinations. If you find that you have made too much juice—as will be the case with the recipes provided—you can simply store the juice for the next day or even freeze them.

Chapter 10:

Mediterranean Diet

What Is It?

Up to this point, we have looked at diets which have been specifically designed around a certain aim. These usually include weight loss or preventing diseases such as heart problems or even type two diabetes. Yet, the Mediterranean diet is not one of these types of diets. It doesn't seek to help weight loss or protect you against heart disease, it just is. The food on this diet was the traditional diet eaten by the people of the Mediterranean region—Greece, Italy, Sicily, etc.—for years before it became a diet that is used by people from around the world. It was during the 1960s that it was noticed that people from these regions were living far healthier lives than those in America or northern Europe (Mayo Clinic Staff, 2019).

After this diet was found, many studies were done on it and it was seen that it promoted weight loss, premature death from heart attacks and other coronary-related deaths, strokes, as well as controlling type 2 diabetes (Gunnars, 2018b). Because of this, the rest of the world started to make use of this diet. Unlike other restrictive diets, the Mediterranean diet only restricts portions of certain foods while cutting out processed and refined foods. There are many ways to follow this diet as long as you stick to the main core of the diet: go as much plant-based as possible while making use of smaller portions of animal products. There is also the promotion of eating healthy fats (Mayo Clinic Staff, 2019). The diet is filled with olives and avocado as well as the oils of these two foods. While red meat is meant to be eaten occasionally, fish is heavily promoted for its healthy fats. Nuts and seeds also contribute to the healthy fats that are eaten on the diet.

Plant-based oils, as well as nuts and seeds, are high in monounsaturated fats. Eating a diet high in these leads to lower total cholesterol as the low-density lipoprotein (LDL) is lowered. Many different kinds of fatty fish, such as salmon, are rich in omega-3 fatty acids (polyunsaturated fat) which helps aid the body in lowering inflammation, decreases triglycerides, as well as reducing blood clotting that can lead to heart attacks and even strokes.

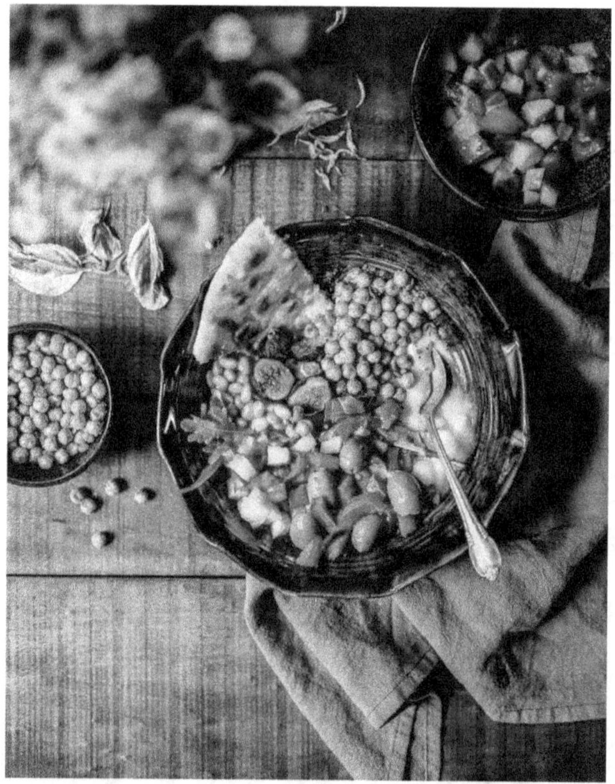

Another thing that sets this diet apart from other diets is that it makes allowance for alcohol. A glass of red wine a day is allowed, if one wants, but is not required. However, if you are a recovering alcoholic or someone who has been told to not drink, then this part of the diet is best to skip.

According to Kris Gunnars (2018b), the best way to understand this diet is that one should eat many fruits, vegetables, and nuts while making use of plant-based oils to cook and add to your foods. Whole grains should be used in all baking as well as when making dishes. Seafood and fish consumption is promoted over poultry, which should be eaten in moderation, and red meat, which should be eaten rarely. Other foods that should be eaten in moderation should be eggs and dairy. All foods that should be cut out include sweet beverages—sodas or fruit juice—any added sugars, all processed meats—sausages or hotdogs—any refined grains or oils, and all processed foods, such as trans fats.

According to the Mayo Clinic Staff (2019), the diet is easy to switch to if you are willing to make a few changes to your eating habits. You need to be consuming between seven and 10 portions of fruits and vegetables a day. Use this opportunity to replace some of your meat-heavy meals with extra portions of vegetables or beans to help you achieve this. Start to cut salt from your diet by making use of different herbs and spices to add flavor to your food. Dairy is important for calcium, but keep it moderate. Try breakfasts with Greek yogurt and fresh fruits. Make use of various fish and seafood up to twice a week that are high in omega-3. Grilling or broiling is best as you want to avoid fried foods on this diet. White bread, rice, pasta, and other refined grains need to go. Switch them out for whole grain varieties which are just as tasty and higher in nutrients and fiber. If you are a fan of bread, cut out the margarine or butter for flavored olive oil mixed with herbs. This diet is so rich in plant-based foods that even vegetarians and vegans can enjoy the benefits from it (Gloeckner, 2019).

Who Can Benefit?

Anyone who wants a non-restrictive, healthy diet where one can still enjoy all the foods that are generally available to you can be rest assured that this diet is for you. Very few food items are on the don't eat list, and it is really only the processed foods that are removed with a suggestion that red meat is eaten in lower doses.

Pros

The advantages of this diet are numerous, as it is backed not only by anecdotal evidence but also scientific evidence (Carroll, 2021). This diet is well-balanced when it comes to nutrition and flavor. It promotes healthy eating which influences your heart health, manages and even prevents type two diabetes, reduces inflammatory markers that are associated with the risk of diabetes, as well as managing one's weight. With the increased fiber as well as good fats, a person feels fuller for longer, so there is no need to snack which can adversely affect your weight. This diet has also been associated with the prevention of cancers such as breast, colon, head, neck, gastric, prostate, as well as liver.

The lifestyle that goes with the Mediterranean diet—people coming together and cooking as a family—has also been proven to do wonders for one's mental state. This lifestyle has been shown to decrease the risk of depressive symptoms in people. With meals that are prepared from scratch, it gives people time to appreciate not only the food but also the people that are working together. This mindset is carried over to the eating part of the meal as well. People who consume their food slowly get more enjoyment from it than those that wolf it down. With eating more fish, there is also an improvement of memory (Gorin, n.d.). This diet is lower in saturated fats in favor of unsaturated fats which is also good for your overall health (Eckelkamp, 2020).

Cons

As good as this diet is, it is very time-consuming to prepare all the meals from scratch (Carroll, 2021). There are also no guidelines in terms of portion or calorie control so this can cause overeating in people who struggle with self-control. As one has to consume dairy in moderation, there may be a lack of calcium or vitamin D if the right foods are not consumed. The diet will need to be reevaluated or supplements made use of.

The diet can also be somewhat costly, especially when it comes to purchases of fish, good olive or avocado oil, as well as nuts and seeds. If possible, buy in bulk or even frozen if available. If someone is already suffering from diabetes, this diet can aggravate it because of the increase of carbohydrates in the fruits and vegetables. It is a good idea to sit with a dietician when it comes to making a decision about which fruits and vegetables should be consumed on the diet.

Processed foods and added sugars are some of the hardest things to give up as they are quite addictive and affordable. Sometimes, they even make up the majority of someone's diet, and thus it becomes very difficult to stop eating them. One may need extra help to move on to this diet if this is the case.

Then there is the promotion of alcohol on the diet. Alcohol in small portions is generally safe for consumption, though many people believe having none is better. It is not as much the alcohol being drunk that is the problem but rather what the person may do after consuming too much alcohol—drunk driving, as an example. This is, however, more based on the person on the diet than the diet itself.

Duration

This is the kind of diet that should be a lifestyle. Not only is the food good for your health, but the culture around the Mediterranean diet is one of teamwork and social interaction (Eckelkamp, 2020). It encourages people to not only work together on the meals but also to enjoy them afterward. Exercise is also encouraged after the large meals. Long walks or hikes are something many Mediterranean people enjoy. If one can afford the lifestyle, then this is a diet that can continue to give many advantages both physically, mentally, and emotionally to those that try it.

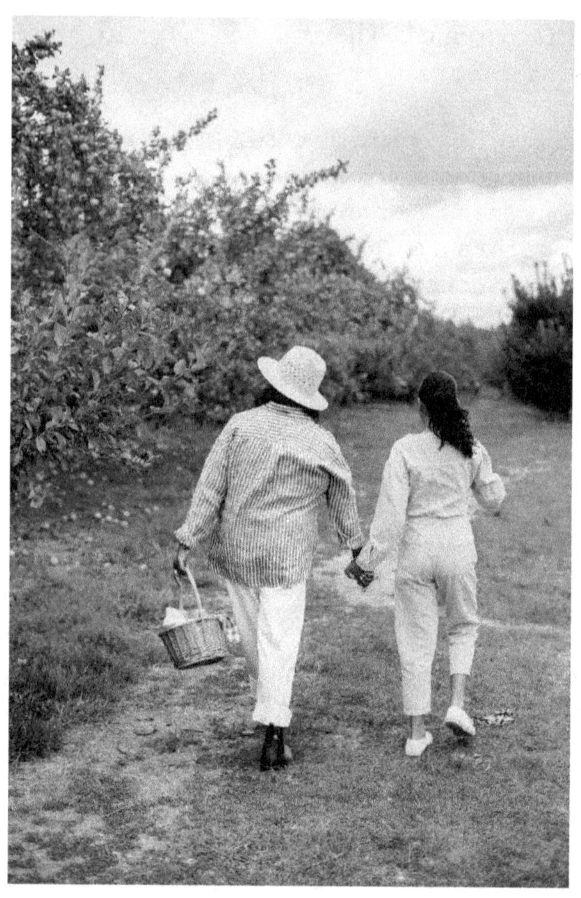

Shopping List

This diet can get a little pricey, so see where you can substitute any of the more expensive items for something less expensive. You do not need to eat salmon when you can get tuna from a can or make use of vegetables or beans to fill your plate with color. Don't be afraid to skip meat completely in favor of plant-based protein meals which are just as good for you. This list was inspired by the works of Kris Gunnars (2018b) and *Olive Tomato* (2018):

- Fresh: There's no limit on the types of fruits and vegetables that one can consume on this diet. You will need many different kinds to fill your plate with up to 10 portions a day, so play around with what you like and don't like. Don't be scared to make use of the starchy vegetables if they are to your taste.

- Dried: Dried olives, tomatoes, and fruit can also make a wonderful addition to your meals.

- Nuts and seeds: All are welcome on the diet, so make use of what your wallet can afford. Sprinkling something like pumpkin or sunflower seeds over a salad is a great way to get a tasty crunch as well as a dose of good fats in your diet.

- Legumes: All are allowed—either cooked, raw, or sprouted you can use.

- Meat: Rarely eat red meat, and eat poultry in moderation. Make sure they are lean cuts of meat. Consume fatty fish and seafood as your main source of meat. Avoid shellfish if you have an allergy to them.

- Dairy: Make use of milk, yogurt, and cheese in moderation. Consider using goat or sheep products when available.

- Eggs: All poultry eggs are welcomed in moderation.

- Baking goods: Avoid added sugar, and bake with whole grains.

- Fats: Plant-based, olive oil, and avocado oil are the most commonly used

- Prepackaged goods: Avoid all processed foods where possible. Canned fish in brine water and canned tomatoes can be used.

- Grains: Whole grains, nothing refined

- Snacks: Stick to fresh fruits and nuts where possible

- Sauces and soups: Make your own sauces and soups with the foods above

- Drinks: Try tea and coffee with no added sugar as well as red wine, which should be limited to one glass or completely avoided.

If you are a vegan or vegetarian, then you are allowed to make use of tofu for this diet as well. Do not skimp on the nuts either, as you will need them for the omega-3 that you cannot get from fish (Hendricks, 2019). If the diet doesn't give you what you need in terms of nutrition, don't be afraid to supplement now and again, but try to broaden your palate by finding foods that give the specific nutrients.

Meal Plan

If you live close to the ocean, it may be significantly easier to get fresh fish than what it is inland, but do make use of canned or frozen fish when possible. Try making some seafood paella, as this is a delicious dish that is well-known on the Mediterranean diet. The ingredients can be found in the frozen food section of most grocers in its own bag. Make sure to have many fruits and vegetables on hand to make your plate colorful and tasty as well. Try to pull the whole family, or several friends, into preparing meals instead of making it one person's responsibility to do everything. Use this time to bond and chat about the day.

The following meal plan was compiled from the works of Kris Gunnars (2018b), Jon Johnson (2019), and Emily Lachtrupp (2020a):

	Breakfast	Lunch	Dinner	Snacks
Day 1	Plain Greek yogurt, berries of choice, and oats.	Two cups of mixed salad greens, cherry tomatoes, and olives. Drizzle a dressing of olive oil and vinegar. Serve with two slices of whole grain bread with two tablespoons of hummus spread on the slices.	A tuna salad, with lots of greens coated in olive oil. Follow with a piece of fruit.	¾ cup raspberries and ¾ cup blackberries.
Day 2	Oatmeal with raisins.	Tuna-spinach salad (one serving).	Whole grain pizza with tomato sauce, low-fat cheese, grilled vegetables, and your choice of lean meat or pine nuts.	Two medium plums and ¾ cup raspberries.
Day 3	Muffin-Tin quiches with	Whole grain sandwich,	One Greek turkey burger	A handful of nuts of

	smoked cheddar and potato (one serving).	with low-fat cheese and fresh vegetables of choice.	with spinach, feta, & tzatziki and a side salad consisting of two cups of mixed greens topped with a tablespoon of vinaigrette.	choice.
Day 4	Healthy pineapple smoothie.	Stuffed sweet potato with a hummus dressing.	Mediterranean lasagna	A cup of cucumber with lemon juice, salt, and pepper to taste and fruit of choice.
Day 5	Plain Greek yogurt with fruits and nuts of choice.	Boiled white beans with spices, laurel, garlic, and cumin with a cup of kale with an olive oil dressing. Top this with tomatoes, cucumber, and feta cheese.	Broiled or grilled salmon, served with brown rice and vegetables of choice.	A ½ cup portion of nonfat plain Greek yogurt with berries of choice.
Day 6	Two eggs scrambled with bell	Roasted vegetables and quinoa	Grilled lamb, with a green salad topped	A medium peach and a medium

	peppers (all colors), onions, and tomatoes. Top your scrambled eggs with a quarter of an avocado.	salad.	with feta, tomatoes, and cucumber with a baked potato on the side.	plum.
Day 7	A slice of whole grain bread with half an avocado and a boiled egg (two if you are hungry).	Prepare a cup of quinoa with bell peppers (all colors), sun-dried tomatoes, and olives. Roast some chickpeas with herbs of choice and add to the mixture. Top everything with some feta or avocado.	Chicken and chickpea soup (one serving).	Some dried fruit and nuts.

The more colorful your plate is, the better it is for you. Stock up on whole grains to enjoy the full benefit of this healthy diet.

Chapter 11:

Military Diet

What Is It?

This is a low-calorie—varying from 1,100 to 1,400 calories a day—low-fat, low-carbohydrate, but high-protein diet that is also known as the three-day diet. This is because the main part of the diet only takes three days and claims to guarantee that you can lose 10 pounds during that time (Crichton-Stuart, 2020). This is not a diet that was designed by the military at all! The name rather comes from the iron willpower and discipline one needs to be able to complete this diet (Military Diet, n.d.). This rapid weight loss program owes this ability to the food combinations that are meant to kick-start your metabolism and burn fat. Even though the calories are very low, this diet doesn't cause the metabolism to slow down because after the three days on the diet, it is followed by four days where one is meant to eat a healthier diet but keeping the calories to about 1,500 (Leech, 2017).

This diet can be repeated for up to a month to allow for about 30 pounds of weight loss (Leech, 2017; Crichton-Stuart, 2020). It is a very good idea to stay hydrated during this time, as when the body is receiving low amounts of calories, it turns to use glycogen stored in the muscles. As we learned with the ketogenic diet, when glycogen is used by the body, a lot of water is lost in the process. It is for this reason that many people believe the loss in weight is more water than fat. There are concerns that the weight will simply return once the diet is over. This is quite possible if one continues to eat more calories than what is necessary. Though, that said, Mayo Clinic Staff (2016a) state that to lose between one and two pounds a week one needs to have a deficit of between 500 and 1,000 calories a day. This puts a person's calorie intake at about 1,500 which is what is suggested for the four days when one gets off of the main part of the diet.

The diet is very simple to follow and the foods are something that almost all grocery store chains will carry. This diet can even be safe for vegans and vegetarians (Leech, 2017). They simply swap out the animal-based foods for foods they can eat. However, they will need to remain within the calorie limits set by the diet.

Who Can Benefit?

As this is a calorie-restrictive diet and not a food group restrictive diet anyone can follow it with ease. One will need to be strict with yourself if you plan on completing this diet, as there is no deviation from what is presented in the meal plan. Excluding trading different foods due to allergies or diet preferences. This is a diet where one can lose weight rapidly so if you are someone that wants to drop a dress or pants size before the weekend then this is something you can try.

Pros

Although this diet is suggested to only be for a short time, there are some benefits to it. It teaches a person to control their calorie intake and limits a large number of processed foods (Crichton-Stuart, 2020). It also promotes the consumption of protein which in turn makes people feel fuller for longer. All of this causes a person to rapidly lose weight during the three days of the military diet. Some even point out that this diet is very similar to intermittent fasting (Leech, 2017). The diet also comes with a structured meal plan that has few deviations from it, so you know exactly what you need to eat and when to eat (Frey, 2021).

Cons

This diet is not suited for the long term (Crichton-Stuart, 2020). If calorie intake is not closely monitored over the four days when one is not on the diet, there is a chance to gain the weight back. It is limited in the nutrients—though this can be rectified with supplements—that are available in the foods you have to eat while on the diet, while what you eat is high in added sugar, salt, and saturated fat. The calorie restriction may also be at a level where a lot of people struggle to do exercise.

Joe Leech (2017) states that with very little vegetables and fruits being eaten, there is too little fiber and thus can cause constipation. There is some promotion of eating junk food in terms of hotdogs as well as ice cream during the three days on the diet. This diet doesn't teach a person to get well but rather only highlights that a person should only cut calories to lose weight and not make an effort to change one's diet for the better (Frey, 2021). The other negatives that once the three days are over, people tend to binge eat due to the calories being too restrictive (Cherney, 2020). This diet is not good for people over the age of 50 who shouldn't be on diets where the calories are limited so severely unless stated so by a medical professional. Counting calories is also rather taxing, especially when one wants to make substitutes for some of the foods on the diet.

Duration

From the disadvantages that are listed, it is very clear that this diet is not a lifestyle choice but should remain as a three-day diet. There is no denying that the diet works well, as lowering the number of calories one eats is a sure way to lose weight. However, extended periods of a low-calorie, low-nutrient diet can cause far more problems than are worth the weight loss. For quick weight loss, this can work, but for long-term results, it is best to choose a diet that can be maintained and turned into a lifestyle.

Shopping List

This is likely the easiest of the diets to shop for as it has a strict guideline that mentions exactly what needs to be eaten on what day and for what meal. Thanks to Cathleen Crichton-Stuart (2020), this shopping list includes foods for the standard military diet as well as vegetarian options:

- Fruit: Grapefruit, banana, and apple (small)

- Vegetables: Green beans, broccoli, and carrots

- Meat: Tuna (in brine) and any red meat that is lean

- Eggs and dairy: Chicken eggs, cottage cheese, and cheddar cheese.

- Grains and bread: Whole grain (for extra fiber)

- Miscellaneous: Peanut butter (sugar-free and salt-free if possible), vanilla ice cream, saltine crackers, hotdog sausages, and stevia if a sweetener is needed

- Drinks: Caffeinated coffee or tea

- Vegan and vegetarian options: Avocado, hummus, tofu, baked beans, unsweetened almond milk, veggie hotdog sausages, dairy-free vanilla ice cream, couscous or quinoa, chickpeas (garbanzo bean), and portobello mushrooms

Possible substitutions for specific portions on this diet were provided by Jennifer Cohen and Cynde Lee (2019).

The calorie value must remain the same when making substitutes:

One slice of bread	One tortilla, or two rice cakes, ⅛ cup of sunflower seeds, ½ high protein bar, ¼ cup yogurt with ½ teaspoon flax seeds, ½ cup whole grain cereal.
Two tablespoons of peanut butter	Two tablespoons of almond, cashew, sunflower seed, soy, or pumpkin butter, two tablespoons sunflower seeds, or two tablespoons of hummus or bean dip.
Coffee and tea	All drinks must be caffeinated. Green tea, sugar-free Red Bull, or sugar-free hot chocolate
½ a can of tuna	To a similar portion (~2.5 ounces), any lean meat (white or red), ½ a can of chickpeas, cheese, tofu, almonds, or ½ an avocado with two tablespoons of hummus
1 cup of green beans	Spinach (or any other dark green leafy vegetable), lettuce, or tomatoes.
½ banana	Grapes, plums, or even applesauce. Or swap for two kiwi fruit, two apricots, or a cup of papaya

1 small apple	Peach, plum, pear, dried apricots, or zucchini
Vanilla ice cream	One cup fruit flavored yogurt, apple juice, flavored almond milk (not chocolate), and dairy-free ice cream (not low-fat)
Egg	One chicken wing, 20 almonds, a cup of milk, $\frac{1}{4}$ cup of nuts or seeds, $\frac{1}{2}$ cup baked beans, or two slices of bacon
One cup of cottage cheese	Ham, cheddar cheese, plain Greek yogurt or ricotta cheese, tofu, or one cup of unsweetened almond milk with two tablespoons of hummus
Five saltine crackers	Rice cakes, couscous, or quinoa
Two hotdogs (~300 calories)	Tofu or soy dogs, bratwurst, turkey dogs, deli meat, beans, lentils, plain tofu, or portobello mushrooms
Broccoli	Spinach, cauliflower, asparagus, or Brussels sprouts
$\frac{1}{2}$ cup carrots	Bell peppers, celery, beets, squash, or parsnip
1 slice of cheddar cheese	Egg, ham, cottage cheese, non-dairy cheese (soy cheese or milk),

	cabbage, or tofu

Even if you aren't a vegetarian or vegan, you can make use of the substitutes for foods that are better suited to your palate and pocket.

Meal Plans

As the substitutes are listed above, they will not be added to the meal plan below. However, the meal plans below will reflect both the standard as well as the vegan and vegetarian options. If you feel that you want to substitute something, consult the table above, and make sure that you remain within your calorie allowance for the day. Remember that whatever drink you decide to add to the diet must be caffeinated, and you must eat the calories suggested for the day. The military meal plans (day one to day three for the standard diet as well as the vegan and vegetarian-friendly option) come from the works of Cathleen Crichton-Stuart (2020) with the calorie values from Joe Leech (2017):

	Breakfast	Lunch	Dinner
Day 1 (1,400 kcal)	One slice of whole wheat toast, half a grapefruit, two tablespoons of peanut butter, (salt and sugar-free), and one cup of coffee or tea.	One slice of toast, half a cup of tuna, one cup of coffee or tea.	Half a banana, three ounces of any lean meat, one cup of green beans, one small apple, and one cup of vanilla ice cream.

Day 2 (1,200 kcal)	One slice of whole wheat toast, one egg (prepared how you want), and half a banana.	One cup of cottage cheese, one hard-boiled egg, and five saltine crackers.	One cup of broccoli. two hotdog sausages, half a banana, half a cup of vanilla ice cream, and half a cup of carrots.
Day 3 (1,100 kcal)	One small apple, five saltine crackers, and a slice of cheddar cheese.	One slice of whole wheat toast and a hard-boiled egg.	Half a banana, one cup of tuna (5 oz), and one cup of vanilla ice cream.

After completing the three days listed above you will need to stick to a diet of 1,500 kcal for a further four days. Below are examples of some 1,500 kcal diets, which include snack options to help you. Remember to keep eating healthy. These suggestions come from the works of Victoria Seaver (2020c) and Diet, Food & Fitness (2019):

	Breakfast	Lunch	Dinner	Snacks
Day 4	Two slices of whole wheat bread, two large eggs, and one tablespoon peanut butter.	One can tuna (in brine), a tablespoon of olive oil mayo for the tuna, two slices of whole grain bread, one tablespoon light dressing for the six	4 oz. grilled chicken (lean), one cheese stick, one cup sweet potato, one cup green beans, one medium apple, and	½ cup fresh pineapple, and ½ cup cottage cheese.

		baby carrots, one cup skim milk, and one slice of low-fat mozzarella cheese.	½ tbsp olive oil spread.	
Day 5	Muesli with raspberries	Chipotle-lime cauliflower taco bowls (one serving).	Mediterranean ravioli with artichokes and olives (one serving).	An ounce of cheddar cheese, one hard-boiled egg, one medium banana, and one tablespoon peanut butter.
Day 6	One hard-boiled egg, ½ cup fat-free cottage cheese, and ½ cup pineapple.	One low-carb wrap, ½ cup bell pepper (green), ½ cup black beans, ¼ avocado, ¼ cup reduced-fat cheddar cheese, two tablespoons tomato salsa, ½ cup shredded lettuce, and one medium peach.	A cup of whole wheat pasta, ½ cup low-sodium marinara sauce, three turkey meatballs, two tablespoons Parmesan cheese, two cups lettuce mix, a tablespoon of olive oil,	20 almonds and a cup of grapes.

			a tbsp balsamic vinegar.	
Day 7	One clementine and baked banana-nut oatmeal cups (2 servings).	Vegetable and hummus sandwich (one serving).	1 serving of Easy salmon cakes over two cups of spinach, and a two-inch piece of whole wheat baguette.	A tablespoon of peanut butter, one medium apple, and a medium banana.

If you still want to lose weight, repeat table one followed by table two until the goal weight is reached. The same practice can be done with the vegan and vegetarian-friendly option below.

	Breakfast	Lunch	Dinner
Day 1 (1,400 kcal)	One slice of whole wheat toast, two tablespoons peanut butter, half a grapefruit, and one cup of coffee or tea.	Two tablespoons of hummus, half an avocado, one cup of coffee or tea, and one slice of whole wheat toast.	One cup of green beans, half a banana, tofu (300 calories), one small apple, one cup of vanilla ice cream (dairy-free if needed).

Day 2 (1,200 kcal)	One slice of whole wheat toast, half a banana, and half a cup of baked beans.	Two tablespoons of hummus, one cup of unsweetened almond milk, five saltine crackers, and half an avocado.	Half a banana, two veggie hotdog sausages, half a cup of carrots, one cup of broccoli, and half a cup of vanilla ice cream (dairy-free if needed).
Day 3 (1,100 kcal)	Half a cup of couscous, 15–20 almonds, and one small apple.	One tablespoon hummus, half an avocado, and one slice of whole wheat bread.	One cup of vanilla ice cream (dairy-free if needed), half a cup of canned chickpeas, and half a banana.

The 1,500 kcal diet plans are courtesy of the works from Victoria Seaver (2020b) and Sara Haas (2016b):

	Breakfast	Lunch	Dinner	Snacks
Day 4	⅓ cup raspberries with one tbsp chopped walnuts over one cup raw oatmeal cooked in two cups of water.	Whole wheat vegetable wrap (one serving), use vegan-friendly cheese.	Mushroom-quinoa vegetable burgers (one serving), use vegan-friendly mayonnaise.	One tablespoon peanut butter, one medium apple, ½ cup low-fat plain Greek yogurt, ¼ cup sliced strawberries, and one tablespoon chia seeds.
Day 5	Maple muesli with banana and almond milk (one serving).	Black bean and mango salad (one serving).	Crispy tofu with edamame and mushroom stir fry (one serving).	Almond-stuffed dates (two servings), guacamole with bell pepper dippers (one serving), and frozen chocolate-coconut milk with strawberries (one serving).

Day 6	One medium apple and one serving of baked banana-nut oatmeal cups.	Lemon-roasted vegetable hummus bowls (one serving).	A two-inch slice of whole wheat baguette with one serving of One-Pot tomato basil pasta with two tablespoons of Parmesan cheese sprinkled on top.	A hard-boiled egg (replace with 20 almonds if vegan), ¼ avocado, a cup of nonfat plain Greek yogurt, ½ cup raspberries, with a tablespoon of chia seeds.
Day 7	One clementine with a serving of avocado and egg toast (replace the egg with 20 almonds if vegan).	Have one serving of curried chickpea stew with a four-inch diameter whole wheat pita.	Beefless vegan tacos (one serving).	A medium apple, ½ cup raspberries, a cup low-fat plain Greek yogurt, a tablespoon of chia seeds, and a tablespoon of peanut butter.

Do not feel limited by what is presented here. As long as your last four days on the military diet contains healthy foods that total to about 1,500 kcal, you can make do with whatever recipes you find online. The most important part is to stick to the calorie count.

Chapter 12:

DASH Diet

What Is It?

The full name of this diet is Dietary Approaches to Stop Hypertension (DASH), and it makes use of dietary choices, rather than medication, to fight hypertension (Mayo Clinic Staff 2016b). The aim of the diet is to increase the number of fruits, vegetables, as well as low-fat dairy options while making moderate use of whole grains, fish, nuts, and poultry to aid in decreasing the level of sodium one eats. On this diet, you will increase your magnesium, calcium, potassium, as well as fiber. The diet actively seeks to encourage people to eat fewer fatty meats, sugar in all forms, full-fat dairy products, sweetened drinks, as well as all forms of sodium, where possible (Oberg, 2020).

This is a diet not designed for losing weight but fighting hypertension, also known as high blood pressure. Weight loss can be experienced on this diet if there are some calorie restrictions as well as adding some exercise. This in itself will also help with lowering blood pressure. High blood pressure is linked to diseases such as heart disease, kidney failure, and even strokes (West, 2018). However, when one makes use of the DASH diet, there are improvements to the body which help with the prevention of certain cancers, heart disease, stroke, osteoporosis, and even aids in preventing type 2 diabetes (Mayo Clinic Staff, 2016b).

High blood pressure is a serious disease and is often referred to as the silent killer (Oberg, 2020). The symptoms generally start as nothing serious where one usually suffers from headaches or even feeling dizzy, which can be signs of many other issues, including dehydration. This is why the symptoms are often overlooked until something far more serious happens such as a stroke or heart attack. The fiber and mineral increases that are seen in the diet often help with imbalances in the body's electrolytes which in turn will cause the body to excrete the excess fluid buildup that can lead to high blood pressure.

Blood pressure is measured at two points, the systolic and the diastolic (West, 2018). Systolic is the blood pressure within the blood vessels as the heart beats, while diastolic is the pressure while the heart is at rest between beats. An average adult's blood pressure should be 120/80 mm Hg—a measurement in millimeters of mercury. If you have a blood pressure reading of anything over 140/90, then you have hypertension and should take steps to control it. The DASH diet aims to lower both the systolic and diastolic by several points in those that have high blood pressure. Although the diet is good for everyone, those that have healthy blood pressure will see very little change in their blood pressure if at all.

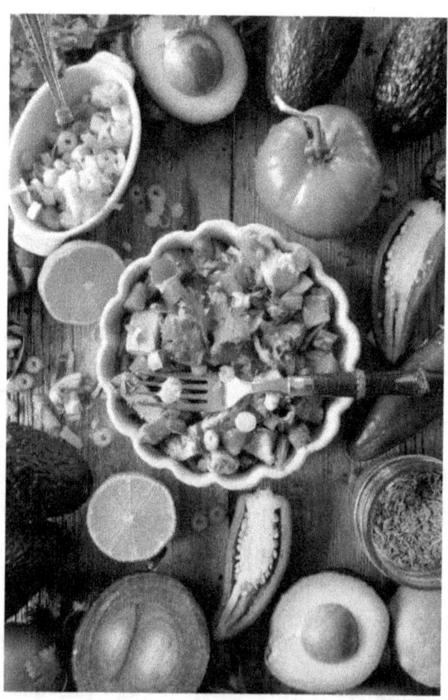

Low sodium doesn't mean boring. A salad can gain flavor with the use of onions, chilis, and lemon juice.

It has been proven that sodium in diets has an effect on one's blood pressure (Mayo Clinic Staff, 2016b). When one looks at the average American diet, the sodium content can be as high as 3,400 mg a day. Salt isn't the only culprit in this. Sodium is often found in ready-made meals, so look at the nutritional label carefully before deciding what you want to eat as a snack next time. The DASH diet has two variants to it. The first is the standard DASH diet when one tries to limit the intake of sodium to about 2,300 mg a day, and the second is the lower sodium DASH diet where the intake of sodium needs to be as low as 1,500 mg per day. This can also be treated as a phase one and phase two if you want to keep lowering your sodium intake over time.

Some people believe that cutting out sodium is good enough to lower one's blood pressure, but you need to be very careful when just cutting out something as important as an electrolyte. Sodium, magnesium, potassium, and calcium are the minerals that help with making sure your muscles work the way they do (WebMD, 2020). Without them, your muscles will cramp and cause pain. So, cutting out one of the minerals without increasing the others can be detrimental to one's health. This is why the DASH diet is so good for those that want to find an effective way to cut down on sodium but not suffer the negatives that could come from it.

A standard DASH diet encourages the following foods (Mayo Clinic Staff, 2016b):

- Grains: Six to eight servings a day—try to concentrate on whole grains, and avoid processed grains (white flour, white bread, etc.).

- Fruits and vegetables: Four to five servings of each a day. You can use either fresh, canned, or frozen, and make use of the edible skins where possible. Remember to wash before consuming.

- Dairy: Two to three servings a day. These need to be kept to low-fat where possible. Be wary of overly processed cheeses that can contain high levels of sodium.

- Meat: Keep to six one-ounce servings a day of red meat, white meat, poultry, and fish—less if you want. Make an effort to trim away all visible fat when possible.

- Legumes, nuts, and seeds: Four to five servings a week. This food type is high in calories, so use them as a snack more than a food source.

- Fats: Keep to about two to three servings a day—less if you can. Make use of unsaturated fats wherever possible.

- Sugar: No more than five servings a week. It can be tough to give up sugar as a whole, so just make use of it less and less until you get to the recommended serving.

- Caffeine: No serving suggestions, but if you have found that caffeine raises your blood pressure, then start limiting your intake.

- Alcohol: Men can have up to two drinks a day while it is suggested that women have no more than one drink a day.

There is no need to immediately jump into this diet unless otherwise stated by a doctor. Start gradually and make small changes to your diet. Something as simple as not adding salt (sodium chloride, also known as common table salt) to your food can make a big improvement in your health. Another change you can do is switch out your regular table salt for something like Himalayan salt (pink Himalayan salt). Although both are salt and contain sodium, the Himalayan salt contains less per gram (368 mg) of it when compared to table salt (381 mg) (Pearson, 2017). It also contains more calcium, potassium, iron, and magnesium.

Who Can Benefit?

As this diet isn't designed for weight loss, it is only really meant for people who are trying to lower their blood pressure naturally without having to rely on medication. This is not to say you can't use this diet to lose weight, but you will have to make use of restricting calories and include exercise to do it.

Pros

The number one advantage of this diet is that it is proved to lower blood pressure through eating less sodium in the diet (Mayo Clinic Staff, 2016b). It is proven not only to see it in people's health, but by various scientific evidence, plus it is backed by institutions like the National Heart, Lung, and Blood Institution as well as the National Institutes of Health (Frey, 2020a). The diet also lowers the risk of diseases such as diabetes, heart diseases, cancer, and metabolic syndrome (West, 2018). There can be weight loss on the diet if exercise is applied as well as controlling the number of calories that are consumed with each meal. As the diet also concentrates on consuming low-fat food items, one's cholesterol is lowered in terms of LDL and triglycerides (My Gut Health Today, 2018).

Malia Frey (2020a) expands on the advantages by saying that this diet is easy to follow as the foods are easily found in all stores, and one doesn't need to buy specialty foods. The diet is quite flexible in terms of calorie consumption, which can be changed depending on whether a person is active or not. With no major food group—carbohydrates, protein, and fats—being avoided, the DASH diet is nutritionally balanced, and you should have no deficiencies in important minerals or vitamins. This diet is designed for controlling blood pressure over a long period and isn't a quick fix, so a lifestyle change is needed to reap all the benefits.

Cons

This is not a diet that is designed for weight loss unless you are willing to put more work into it other than just a food change (Mayo Clinic Staff, 2016b). One of the biggest complaints is that this diet lacks taste due to cutting salt from the diet (Oberg, 2020). Salt is but one flavor that you can make use of when cooking. There are an array of spices and herbs that are used to give more taste than salt ever could. Teaching yourself how to make use of these flavor enhancers will change the way you see and taste food once you give up salt.

This is not a short-term diet and needs to be made into a lifestyle change if you want to avoid the diseases that are associated with hypertension (My Gut Health Today, 2018). Most people are addicted to the taste of salt, and it is for this reason that the diet can be difficult to maintain (Frey, 2020a). Not only that but one has to give up all foods that are labeled as a convenience, such as protein bars, microwave dinners, store-bought smoothies, etc. These food types are generally far too high in sodium to be allowed on the DASH diet.

Sadly, unlike many other diets, though DASH has many online resources one can make use of, there are very few, if any, support groups to help those that are trying the diet for the first time. Diets can be completed or given up depending on how much support one gets when trying to complete them, so this could negatively affect someone that requires support. This diet isn't for everyone, especially if you are a person who has to take renin—as a form of treatment of hypertension. You will need to have a doctor's go-ahead to try this diet. The diet may also have to be modified for people who suffer from uncontrolled type 2 diabetes, chronic heart failure, celiac disease, as well as lactose intolerance. Though a small restriction, giving up salt and sugar at the same time is quite a chore for most people and leads to some people not even willing to try the diet, rather going the route of medical intervention.

Duration

To avoid the silent killer that hypertension is, you will have to make a lifestyle change. It isn't just about cutting sodium from your diet but also making the choice to avoid prepackaged and other convenience foods. It is cutting out sweets, high-fat dairy products, and considering getting more exercise in. The DASH diet isn't something that can be followed for a few weeks to fix a problem and then you can go back to the way you used to eat. No, to ensure that your blood pressure is controlled before having to have a medical intervention, it is a good idea to make this diet part of your life.

Even if you are a healthy individual with no history of blood pressure issues, it is not a bad idea to cut back on highly processed foods in favor of fresh fruits, vegetables, and whole grains. There is nothing to lose and everything to gain.

Shopping List

The very first thing that needs to be removed from your shopping cart is the replacement of the empty saltshaker. After that, you will need to place back all those prepackaged meals. However, before you do, have a look at the nutritional label and realize just how much sodium is actually in the food that we consume daily. It will shock you! The following shopping list was designed using the works of *Berkeley Life* (2017) and James Waygood (2019):

- Fruits: All berries, citrus (check to make sure it doesn't clash with any medications), stone fruit, pineapples, apples, pears, mangoes, grapes, kiwis, etc.

- Vegetables: Always go for dark green, leafy vegetables then add color with peppers, beets, tomatoes, legumes, potatoes, sweet potatoes, onions, broccoli, cauliflower, etc.

- Protein: Lean meats—all kinds—and eggs

- Dairy: Stick to low-fat wherever you can, and avoid the sweetened options as seen with yogurt. Keep to moderation.

- Nuts and seeds: Make use of as many different kinds but make sure they are not salted. Pumpkin seed, sunflower seeds, hazelnuts, almonds, etc.

- Fats: Any unsaturated fats will work well with this diet. Coconut oil, olive oil, and avocado oil

- Prepackaged goods: No, don't even look at it. Avoid at all costs.

- Grains: Whole grains, avoid all refined grains as they will contain more sodium. Whole wheat bread and pasta, brown rice, barley, quinoa, etc.

- Snacks: Homemade popcorn, low-fat, low-sugar chocolate (high cocoa value)

- Sauces and soups: Anything that isn't homemade should be avoided as more canned or prepackaged goods will have a high level of sodium. If canned goods cannot be avoided, then look for low-sodium options.

- Sugar: Sugar is allowed on the diet but should be heavily restricted. Honey, agave syrup, etc.

- Herbs and spices: Chili powder, cumin, garlic powder, oregano, onion powder, parsley, pepper (black and white), cayenne pepper, garlic, paprika, mint, etc. (The Best DASH Diet

Recipes, 2019). Some premade mixtures can be bought, but do keep an eye on their sodium content.

If making use of baked goods, be wary that there is sodium present. Each type of bread will have different sodium amounts. If you want to make use of this food source, it is a good idea to know how to read a food label. If you are a vegan or vegetarian that has a problem with high blood pressure, you can follow this diet quite easily by just removing the animal-based products you do not want to consume.

Meal Plan

The first step to completing this meal plan is to make sure that you are not adding any extra salt but rather experimenting with the various herbs and spices that are available to you. Herbs and spices are not your only go-to when it comes to flavor. Look at using various vegetables to flavor soups, or make your own stocks instead of buying from the store. The meal plan was designed using the works of Helen West (2018), Mayo Clinic staff (2018), and Victoria Seaver (2020a):

	Breakfast	Lunch	Dinner	Snacks
Day 1	A whole wheat bagel with two tablespoons of peanut butter (salt-free), a medium orange, a cup of fat-free milk.	Two cups mixed lettuce, ¼ cup grated carrot, ½ cup cucumber, and two tablespoons vinaigrette. Add to ½ large whole wheat pita	Six ounces of cod fillet, a cup of mashed potatoes (no salt added), ½ cup of green peas, and ½ cup of broccoli.	A pear dusted with cinnamon and ¾ cup raspberries.

		round with ¼ cup hummus.		
Day 2	A cup of oatmeal with a cup of skim milk, ½ cup of blueberries, and ½ cup of freshly squeezed orange juice.	Make a salad with four cups of fresh spinach leaves, one pear, ½ cup orange sections, ⅓ cup chopped almonds, add two tablespoons vinaigrette. Add 12 wheat crackers (low-salt) and a cup of fat-free milk.	1 ½ cups Chicken chili with sweet potatoes with ¼ avocado and a tablespoon nonfat plain Greek yogurt. Enjoy a medium plum for dessert.	1 medium orange, 4 whole grain crackers with 1 ½ ounces of cottage cheese, and ½ cup of fresh pineapple.
Day 3	⅔ cup nonfat plain Greek yogurt topped with five dried figs, two teaspoons chia seeds, and a light drizzle of honey.	Two slices of whole grain bread, a tablespoon mayonnaise, 1 ½ cups of green salad, and three ounces of canned tuna (low-salt).	Grill a four-ounce cod and serve with ½ cup brown rice with steamed green vegetables of choice. Add a small sourdough roll with a cup of fresh berries with chopped mint and an	A cup of grapes and two clementines.

			herbal iced tea.	
Day 4	A cup of fresh fruits of choice, topped with a cup of plain Greek low-fat yogurt and ⅓ cup almonds. Enjoy together with a bran muffin and a cup of fat-free milk.	Add two cups of mixed greens, ¾ cup chopped vegetables, such as cucumber and cherry tomatoes, ⅓ cup canned white beans, and ½ avocado. Toss vegetables together with two tablespoons of vinaigrette.	A three-ounce serving of lean chicken breast cooked with a tsp of vegetable oil, ½ cup of both broccoli and carrots, and a cup of brown rice.	A cup of fat-free, low-calorie yogurt with four vanilla wafers.
Day 5	A slice of whole wheat bread, one egg fried in ¼ tsp olive oil, and a medium banana.	A medium whole wheat tortilla filled with three ounces of cooked chicken and ½ cup apple (chopped), with 1 ½ tablespoons light mayonnaise and ½	Curried cauliflower steaks with rice and tzatziki (one serving) and for dessert one serving of Chocolate and nut butter bites.	A cup of low-fat yogurt, a medium apple, and a medium banana.

		teaspoon curry powder for taste. On the side, have eight baby carrots and a cup of fat-free milk.		
Day 6	Two boiled eggs, two slices of turkey bacon with ½ cup of baked beans (low-salt), ½ cup of tomatoes, and two slices of whole wheat toast. Enjoy with ½ cup of freshly squeezed orange juice.	Vegetable and hummus sandwich.	A cup cooked whole wheat spaghetti with a cup marinara sauce, add two cups mixed salad greens with a tablespoon low-fat Caesar dressing. Enjoy with a small whole wheat roll and a nectarine.	A clementine and ½ cup of grapes.
Day 7	Peanut-butter cinnamon toast (one serving).	Two slices of whole wheat bread, three ounces of lean chicken, ½ cup of green salad, 1	Lemon-Herb salmon with caponata and farro.	Home-made trail mix consisting of ¼ cup raisins. 22 unsalted mini

		½ ounces of low-fat cheese, and ½ cup tomatoes.		pretzels, and two tablespoons sunflower seeds.

Do not add any salt to anything you are cooking or preparing on this diet. When using canned goods, make sure to check the sodium content or make use of the light version. If possible, switch out canned goods for fresh. Experiment with herbs and spices to bring out the natural flavors of food instead of reaching for the saltshaker.

Conclusion

Whether you are an aspiring athlete or someone who spends hours in front of a computer for work, your diet is important. Your body is unable to do what you need of it if you do not give it the fuel it requires. Whether that fuel is obtained from the classic glycolysis metabolic system or through a ketosis metabolic system is completely up to you. A diet is something that is not only what a doctor may prescribe for a certain condition—epilepsy, high blood pressure, or even type 2 diabetes—but is also deeply personal to the person trying it.

A diet is so much more than just food; sometimes a person chooses what they eat based on culture or preference of certain types of food as in the case of vegans and vegetarians. While some people who want to lose weight quickly opt to change their metabolic process completely by cutting out a whole group of macromolecules, such as carbohydrates in terms of the ketogenic and Atkins diet. Other people prefer to keep their calorie intake below 1,500 calories a day to have the pounds melt away even quicker, as with the military diet.

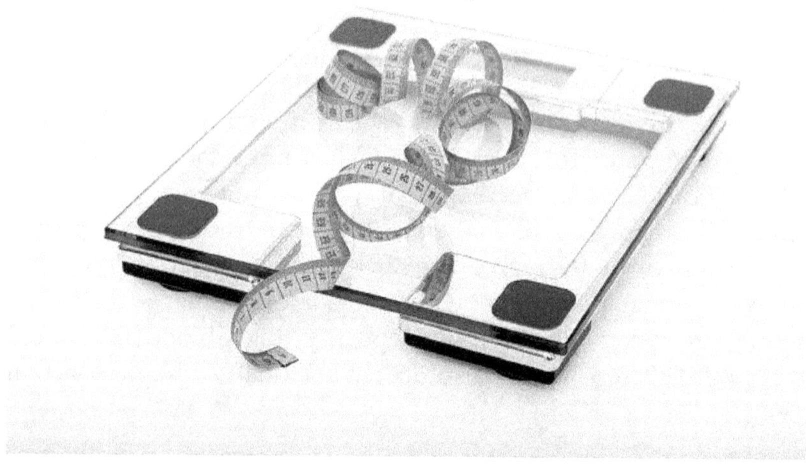

The scale doesn't define who you are! Eat healthy to discover who you are.

There is no denying that irrespective of which diet a person attempts, most people do it as a way to lose weight and to try and stay healthy. As to which diet is the best, well that is up to you to decide, as each of the diets discussed comes with its own advantages and disadvantages, some of which can be more detrimental than good for you. Some diets are meant to be for the short term—a few days to a week maximum—while others expect you to be able to change your entire life to maintain them. The results of these lifestyle changes are not instantaneous—although some of us wish it to be so—and it takes weeks to months to see the results of your hard work. Some of the diets are significantly cheaper to maintain while others can get to be a little pricey.

What is the price tag on health worth? Eating a well-balanced meal every day improves your quality of life in so many ways. Yet, with most of the diets, suggesting that processed and prepackaged food should be given up, this means that you will be in charge of cooking your own meals every single day. This is a little tough on a person who is busy with work and family life. Yet, if a little time is taken to draw the whole family together to help with diet choices, shopping, and even creating wonderful meals, this will not become a chore. As seen with the Mediterranean diet, it isn't just about the food but about the community of people that prepare the meals. If we can take what is taught in the culture of the Mediterranean people and apply it to all of the diets, it will make it easier to stick to creating wonderful meals, irrespective of which diet you choose.

Even the diets that should only be maintained for several days have their benefits. So, before you look into starting a diet, think about what you want from it. Are you trying to identify a food allergy? Lose weight? Build muscle? There are diets, many not even discussed in this book, which can help you achieve your dreams. However, it takes work. Either through research, preparing a shopping list, or preparing meals for days in advance. Don't think that you can just jump into a diet to try it. This is where the disadvantages will hit you the hardest. If you want to get the most from your chosen diet, you need to be prepared to do the work, do the research, and most of all, be ready for the transformation you will undergo as you make this journey. Starting a journey alone can be tough, but it is possible, but if you want extra help, why not get your family or friends to join in with you? That way you can help each other prepare meals, talk about your changes, and recognize when someone is being affected by the disadvantages so that you can help them to get right back on track.

So, make the change today. You have all the knowledge at your fingertips. With shopping lists, meal plans, and all the advantages and disadvantages in this book, you can make a choice right now to no longer be trapped in the body you no longer want. You can make the change, but it starts one day at a time. Trade out your processed meals for some good old fashion fruits and vegetables and get ready to prepare the meals of a lifetime to get the body and health that you deserve today. If you feel that you have learned something of value in this book, don't hesitate to tell your friends and family so that they too can join in the body transformation of a lifetime through sticking to a diet of choice.

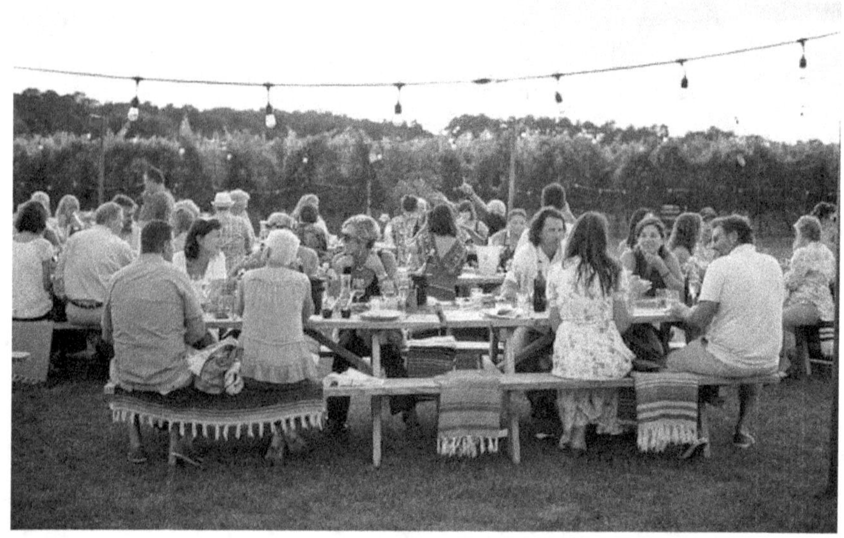

A diet isn't just about food. It truly is a lifestyle change. It is something anyone can do if they put their mind to it. The more support you have, the easier it will be.

References

A Good Hue. (2013, September 27). *How to: 3 day DIY juice cleanse with shopping list.* https://agoodhueblog.com/2013/09/how-to-3-day-diy-juice-cleanse-with-shopping-list/

Alena. (2017, April 26). *15 different types of vegan diets: Which is right for you?* Nutriciously. https://nutriciously.com/different-vegan-diets/

All Day I Dream About Food. (2017a, March 9). *Low carb Mexican cauliflower rice.* https://alldayidreamaboutfood.com/low-carb-mexican-cauliflower-rice/

All Day I Dream About Food. (2017b, November 17). *Low carb butter pecan cookies.* https://alldayidreamaboutfood.com/low-carb-butter-pecan-cookies-2/

All Day I Dream About Food. (2018a, January 11). *Sheet pan chicken and vegetables.* https://alldayidreamaboutfood.com/keto-sheet-pan-chicken/

All Day I Dream About Food. (2018b, July 8). *Asian steak bites - easy keto recipe.* https://alldayidreamaboutfood.com/easy-steak-bites/

All Day I Dream About Food. (2018c, October 6). *Low carb cinnamon crunch cereal.* https://alldayidreamaboutfood.com/cinnamon-crunch-cereal-and-paying-it-forward/

All Day I Dream About Food. (2019a, February 26). *Cheesy chicken broccoli casserole - keto recipe.* https://alldayidreamaboutfood.com/cheesy-chicken-broccoli-casserole/

All Day I Dream About Food. (2019b, June 16). *Keto sheet pan pancakes.* https://alldayidreamaboutfood.com/keto-sheet-pan-pancakes/

All Day I Dream About Food. (2020, January 7). *Easy keto meal plan for beginners.* https://alldayidreamaboutfood.com/easy-keto-meal-plan/

Anderson, J. (2020, November 19). *What is the zone diet?* Verywell Fit. https://www.verywellfit.com/the-zone-diet-4769505

Ansel, K. (2017, February). *Curried cauliflower steaks with red rice & tzatziki.* EatingWell. https://www.eatingwell.com/recipe/256510/curried-cauliflower-steaks-with-red-rice-tzatziki/

Aobadia, A. (2021a, March 9). *Dairy-Free keto latte - quick breakfast recipe.* Diet Doctor. https://www.dietdoctor.com/recipes/keto-dairy-free-latte

Aobadia, A. (2021b, March 19). *Cheesy mexican keto quesadillas (5g net carb).* Diet Doctor. https://www.dietdoctor.com/recipes/keto-quesadillas

Aobadia, A. (2021c, March 20). *Keto pizza - the best pizza recipe ever with video.* Diet Doctor. https://www.dietdoctor.com/recipes/keto-pizza

Aobadia, A. (2021d, March 22). *Keto Meat Pie with Cheese & Crust (6g carb).* Diet Doctor. https://www.dietdoctor.com/recipes/keto-meat-pie

Aobadia, A. (2021e, March 22). *Keto spinach frittata — breakfast recipe.* Diet Doctor. https://www.dietdoctor.com/recipes/keto-frittata-fresh-spinach

Aobadia, A. (2021f, March 23). *Keto pesto & feta chicken casserole — recipe* (video). Diet Doctor. https://www.dietdoctor.com/recipes/keto-pesto-chicken-casserole

Aobodia, A. (2021a, March 18). *Keto Avocado, Bacon & goat-cheese salad - recipe.* Diet Doctor. https://www.dietdoctor.com/recipes/avocado-bacon-goat-cheese-salad

Aobodia, A. (2021b, March 29). *Keto pancakes with berries and cream - recipe.* Diet Doctor. https://www.dietdoctor.com/recipes/keto-pancakes-berries-whipped-cream

Aobodia, A. (2021c, March 30). *Keto baked bacon omelet with spinach — recipe.* Diet Doctor. https://www.dietdoctor.com/recipes/keto-baked-bacon-omelet

Atkins. (n.d.-a). *List of low carb foods for Atkins 20, phase 1.* Retrieved March 25, 2021, from https://www.atkins.com/how-it-works/atkins-20/phase-1/low-carb-foods

Atkins. (n.d.-b). *The Atkins grocery list for low carb dieting.* Retrieved March 25, 2021, from https://www.atkins.com/how-it-works/library/articles/stock-your-kitchen-with-atkins-low-carb-grocery-list

Atkins. (n.d.-c). *Your phase 1 (week 1) meal planner 20g of carbohydrates per day* [PDF]. Atkins. Retrieved April 1, 2021, from https://sa.atkins.com/mealplans.html

Atkins. (n.d.-d). *Your phase 1 meal (week 2) planner 20g of carbohydrates per day* [PDF]. Atkins. Retrieved April 1, 2021, from https://sa.atkins.com/mealplans.html

Atkins. (n.d.-e). *Your phase 2 meal planner (week 1) 25g of carbohydrates per day* [PDF]. Retrieved April 1, 2021, from https://sa.atkins.com/mealplans.html

Atkins. (n.d.-f). *Your phase 2 meal planner (week w) 25g of carbohydrates per day* [PDF]. Retrieved April 1, 2021, from https://sa.atkins.com/mealplans.html

Atkinson, L. (2011, November 6). *The dukan diet meal plan.* Body and Soul. https://www.bodyandsoul.com.au/diet/diets/the-dukan-diet-meal-plan/news-story/b9b1ef0306bba3d7dcd7decd607e92f2

Bandurski, K. (2021, February 2). *The ultimate 7-day vegetarian meal plan for anyone trying to eat less meat.* Taste of Home. https://www.tasteofhome.com/collection/vegetarian-meal-plan/

Berkeley Life. (2017, September 22). *Shopping list: DASH diet foods.* https://www.berkeleylife.com/wellness/functional-foods/shopping-list-dash-diet-foods/

Berry Abundant Life. (n.d.). *Raw vegan food list.* Retrieved March 27, 2021, from https://www.berryabundantlife.com/complete-raw-vegan-food-list/

Better Health USA. (2007, October 8). *Rating the Atkins diet: Advantages and disadvantages.* https://www.betterhealthusa.com/public/250.cfm

Bonom, D. (2016). *Chicken chili with sweet potatoes.* EatingWell. https://www.eatingwell.com/recipe/255168/chicken-chili-with-sweet-potatoes/

Boston Medical Center. (n.d.). *Nutrition and weight management.* Boston Medical Center. Retrieved March 23, 2021, from https://www.bmc.org/nutrition-and-weight-management/weight-management

Brazier, Y. (2020a, January 20). *What to know about the vegetarian diet.* Medical News Today. https://www.medicalnewstoday.com/articles/8749

Brazier, Y. (2020b, January 29). *The zone diet: All you need to know.* Www.medicalnewstoday.com. https://www.medicalnewstoday.com/articles/7382

Brazier, Y. (2020c, April 24). *Dukan diet: Phases, cooking ideas, and effectiveness.* Www.medicalnewstoday.com. https://www.medicalnewstoday.com/articles/219612

Brazier, Y. (2020d, April 27). *The raw food diet: Types, benefits, and risks.* Www.medicalnewstoday.com. https://www.medicalnewstoday.com/articles/7381

Brown, J. (2020, January 23). *Are there health benefits to going vegan?* Bbc.com. https://www.bbc.com/future/article/20200122-are-there-health-benefits-to-going-vegan

Cadry, N. (2020, June 2). *Creamy cashew salad dressing (vegan).* Cadry's Kitchen. https://cadryskitchen.com/cashew-dressing/#wprm-recipe-container-29592

Campbell, K. (2019, August 28). *Peanut butter cup chaffles.* That Low Carb Life. https://thatlowcarblife.com/peanut-butter-cup-chaffles/

Carroll, C. (2021, March 25). *Is the Mediterranean diet a healthier way for you to eat?* Verywell Fit. https://www.verywellfit.com/the-mediterranean-diet-pros-and-cons-4685664

Casner, C. (2017, February). *Muffin-Tin quiches with smoked cheddar & potato.* EatingWell. https://www.eatingwell.com/recipe/256433/muffin-tin-quiches-with-smoked-cheddar-potato/

Casner, C. (2018, October). *Cinnamon roll overnight oats.* EatingWell. https://www.eatingwell.com/recipe/268775/cinnamon-roll-overnight-oats/

Casner, C. (2019a, March). *One-Pot tomato basil pasta.* EatingWell. https://www.eatingwell.com/recipe/270915/one-pot-tomato-basil-pasta/

Casner, C. (2019b, March). *Skillet lemon chicken & potatoes with kale.* EatingWell.

https://www.eatingwell.com/recipe/272467/skillet-lemon-chicken-potatoes-with-kale/

Casner, C. (2019c, June). *Baked banana-nut oatmeal cups.* EatingWell. https://www.eatingwell.com/recipe/274166/baked-banana-nut-oatmeal-cups/

Centoni, D. (n.d.). *Roasted cauliflower & potato curry soup.* EatingWell. Retrieved April 3, 2021, from https://www.eatingwell.com/recipe/256519/roasted-cauliflower-potato-curry-soup/

Cherney, K. (2020, January 21). *The military diet: A review and beginner's guide of the 3-day plan.* EverydayHealth.com. https://www.everydayhealth.com/diet-and-nutrition/diet/military-diet-review-beginners-guide-day-plan/

Chocolate Covered Katie. (2018, July 23). *Fat bombs (keto, vegan, no bake).* https://chocolatecoveredkatie.com/fat-bombs-recipe-keto/

Clarke, C. (2020, September 13). *Comprehensive guide: Vegetarian keto diet [recipes & meal plan].* Ruled Me. https://www.ruled.me/comprehensive-guide-vegetarian-ketogenic-diet/

Clean Program. (2019a, June 26). *The bright lentil beet salad you'll make on repeat.* https://blog.cleanprogram.com/lentil-beet-salad/

Clean Program. (2019b, September 18). *You can make these easy vegan summer rolls anytime.* https://blog.cleanprogram.com/summer-rolls/

Clean Program. (2020a, February 26). *Vegan breakfast hash.* https://blog.cleanprogram.com/vegan-breakfast/

Clean Program. (2020b, July 1). *This lentil burger is a recipe for backyard fun.* https://blog.cleanprogram.com/lentil-burger/

Clean Program. (2020c, October 14). *Yummy vegan carrot tempeh sandwich.* https://blog.cleanprogram.com/tempeh-sandwich/

Clean Program. (n.d.). *Pre-cleanse meal archives.* Retrieved April 2, 2021, from https://blog.cleanprogram.com/category/meal/

Cohen, J., & Lee, C. (2019, December 11). *The 3 day military diet meal plan and menu for weight loss.* MedicineNet. https://www.medicinenet.com/the_3_day_military_diet/article .htm

Crichton-Stuart, C. (2020, January 6). *What is the military diet and does it work?* Www.medicalnewstoday.com. https://www.medicalnewstoday.com/articles/323952

Cultures for Health. (n.d.). *How to make raw milk yogurt | raw milk yogurt recipes.* Retrieved April 3, 2021, from https://www.culturesforhealth.com/learn/yogurt/raw-milk-yogurt/

Dansinger, M. (2021, February 7). *Low-Fat diets for weight loss.* WebMD https://www.webmd.com/women/reducing-dietary-fat

Dansky, L. (2020, July). *Turkey & sweet potato chili.* EatingWell. https://www.eatingwell.com/recipe/280946/turkey-sweet-potato-chili/

Diet Doctor. (2015, July 23). *Low carb and keto made simple.* https://www.dietdoctor.com/

Diet, Food & Fitness. (2019, March 20). *Your 3-day heart-healthy meal plan: 1,500 calories.* Health Essentials from Cleveland Clinic. https://health.clevelandclinic.org/your-3-day-heart-healthy-meal-plan-1500-calories/

Doheny, K. (2019, November 4). *Are there health downsides to vegetarian diets?* WebMDhttps://www.webmd.com/diet/obesity/news/201911 04/are-there-health-downsides-to-vegetarian-diets

Dolsan, L. (2021, March 18). *What is the dukan diet? Pros, cons, and what you can eat.* Verywell Fit. https://www.verywellfit.com/dukan-diet-review-2242251

Down to Earth. (2020, March 5). *Top 10 Reasons for Going Veggie.* Down to Earth Organic and Natural. https://www.downtoearth.org/go-veggie/top-10-reasons

Dr. Sears' Zone Labs. (n.d.). *Zone body fat calculator.* Retrieved March 26, 2021, from https://zonediet.com/resources/body-fat-calculator/?AID=10552992&PID=100090071&SID=41977X1601025Xe9a0bca1c22d0d39dbedc83658a76a3a&utm_source=CJ&utm_medium=affiliate&cjevent=1c09a1538e2411eb818200510a180511

Drugs.com. (2020, March 4). *Low fat diet.* https://www.drugs.com/cg/low-fat-diet.html

Dukan Diet.com. (n.d.). *Dukan diet food list - 100 allowed foods.* Weight Loss Diet Plan & Coaching - Dukan Diet. Retrieved March 27, 2021, from https://www.dukandiet.com/low-carb-diet/food-list

Eating Well Test Kitchen. (2004). *Easy salmon cakes.* EatingWell. https://www.eatingwell.com/recipe/248780/easy-salmon-cakes/

Eating Well Test Kitchen. (2016, February). *Falafel salad with lemon-tahini dressing.* EatingWell. https://www.eatingwell.com/recipe/253015/falafel-salad-with-lemon-tahini-dressing/

Eckelkamp, S. (2020, December 5). *Pros & cons of the Mediterranean diet.* OliveOil.com. https://www.oliveoil.com/mediterranean-diet-pros-cons/

Editor. (2019, January 15). *Types of ketogenic diet.* Diabetes. https://www.diabetes.co.uk/keto/types-of-ketogenic-diet.html

Eenfeldt, A. (2021a, January 26). *Fruits and berries: A keto guide.* Diet Doctor. https://www.dietdoctor.com/low-carb/keto/fruits

Eenfeldt, A. (2021b, March 7). *Keto vegetables – the visual guide to the best and worst.* Diet Doctor. https://www.dietdoctor.com/low-carb/keto/vegetables

Eenfeldt, A. (2021c, March 30). *14-Day keto meal plan with recipes & shopping lists.* Diet Doctor. https://www.dietdoctor.com/low-carb/keto/diet-plan/u3

Elcowgirl. (n.d.). *Vegan bacon recipe.* Www.food.com. Retrieved April 3, 2021, from https://www.food.com/recipe/vegan-bacon-148899

Epperson, S. (2019, November). *Slow-Cooker Mediterranean stew.* EatingWell. https://www.eatingwell.com/recipe/277511/slow-cooker-mediterranean-stew/

Evans, K. M. (2021, March 9). *The best slow-cooked bone broth 3 ways.* Diet Doctor. https://www.dietdoctor.com/recipes/bone-broth

Fogoros, R. N. (2021, March 24). *What is a low-fat diet?* Verywell Health. https://www.verywellhealth.com/low-fat-diets-and-the-heart-1746349

Frey, M. (2020a, January 17). *Pros and cons of the DASH diet.* Verywell Fit. https://www.verywellfit.com/dash-diet-pros-and-cons-3973825

Frey, M. (2020b, November 30). *Pros and cons of a juice diet.* Verywell Fit. https://www.verywellfit.com/juice-diets-for-weight-loss-3495297

Frey, M. (2020c, December 2). *Pros and cons of a vegetarian diet.* Verywell Fit. https://www.verywellfit.com/vegetarian-diet-pros-and-cons-4770717

Frey, M. (2021, March 11). *What is the 3-day military diet?* Verywell Fit. https://www.verywellfit.com/the-3-day-military-diet-review-3495299

Gavin, M. L. (2018, February). *Figuring out fat and calories.* Kidshealth.org. https://kidshealth.org/en/teens/fat-calories.html

Gloeckner, C. (2019, November 6). *Vegan mediterranean diet plan.* EatingWell. https://www.eatingwell.com/article/2058271/vegan-mediterranean-diet-plan/

Gorin, A. (n.d.). *What are the pros and cons of the Mediterranean diet?* Food Network. Retrieved March 29, 2021, from https://www.foodnetwork.com/healthy/articles/mediterranean-diet-pros-cons

Gunnars, K. (2018a, March 27). *Do low-fat diets really work?* Healthline. https://www.healthline.com/nutrition/do-low-fat-diets-work

Gunnars, K. (2018b, July 24). Mediterranean diet 101: A meal plan and beginner's guide. Healthline. https://www.healthline.com/nutrition/mediterranean-diet-meal-plan

Gunnars, K. (2018c, August 2). *The Atkins diet: Everything you need to know.* Healthline. https://www.healthline.com/nutrition/atkins-diet-101

Haas, S. (2016a, April). Mediterranean tuna-spinach salad. EatingWell. https://www.eatingwell.com/recipe/251355/mediterranean-tuna-spinach-salad/

Haas, S. (2016b, August 4). *1-Day 1,500-calorie vegan meal plan.* EatingWell. https://www.eatingwell.com/article/289030/1-day-1500-calorie-vegan-meal-plan/

Haas, S. (2016c, August). *Almond-Stuffed dates.* EatingWell. https://www.eatingwell.com/recipe/254638/almond-stuffed-dates/

Haas, S. (2016d, August). *Black bean & mango salad.* EatingWell. https://www.eatingwell.com/recipe/254639/black-bean-mango-salad/

Haas, S. (2016e, August). *Crispy tofu with black rice & edamame-mushroom stir-fry.* EatingWell. https://www.eatingwell.com/recipe/254636/crispy-tofu-with-black-rice-edamame-mushroom-stir-fry/

Haas, S. (2016f, August). *Frozen chocolate-coconut milk with strawberries.* EatingWell. https://www.eatingwell.com/recipe/254641/frozen-chocolate-coconut-milk-with-strawberries/

Haas, S. (2016g, August). *Guacamole with bell pepper dippers.* EatingWell. https://www.eatingwell.com/recipe/254640/guacamole-with-bell-pepper-dippers/

Haas, S. (2016h, August). *Maple granola.* EatingWell. https://www.eatingwell.com/recipe/254637/maple-granola/

Haas, S. (2020). *Sheet-Pan salmon with sweet potatoes & broccoli.* EatingWell. https://www.eatingwell.com/recipe/281181/sheet-pan-salmon-with-sweet-potatoes-broccoli/

Haas, S. (n.d.). *Peanut butter & chia berry jam English muffin.* EatingWell. Retrieved April 3, 2021, from https://www.eatingwell.com/recipe/255160/peanut-butter-chia-berry-jam-english-muffin/

Hanuise, P. (n.d.). *Rainbow salad [vegan].* One Green Planet. Retrieved April 3, 2021, from https://www.onegreenplanet.org/vegan-recipe/rainbow-salad/

Hartney, E. (2020, November 18). *How addictive is sugar really?* Verywell Mind. https://www.verywellmind.com/sugar-addiction-22149

Hay, D. (2021, March 21). *A 30-day juicing challenge (+ 3 favorite juice recipes).* No Meat Athlete. https://www.nomeatathlete.com/30-day-juice-challenge/

Health.gov. (n.d.). *Current dietary guidelines.* Retrieved March 23, 2021, from https://health.gov/our-work/food-nutrition/current-dietary-guidelines

Hendley, J. (2019a). *Curried chickpea stew.* EatingWell. https://www.eatingwell.com/recipe/270561/curried-chickpea-stew/

Hendley, J. (2019b, May). *Apple & peanut butter toast.* EatingWell. https://www.eatingwell.com/recipe/272745/apple-peanut-butter-toast/

Hendricks, S. (2019, January 18). *7 foods you can eat if you're a vegan and on the Mediterranean diet.* Insider. https://www.insider.com/mediterranean-vegan-diet-foods-2019-1

Hodges, C. (2019, October). *Chipotle-Lime cauliflower taco bowls.* EatingWell. https://www.eatingwell.com/recipe/276890/chipotle-lime-cauliflower-taco-bowls/

Hodges, C. A. (2019a, June). *Mediterranean ravioli with artichokes & olives.* EatingWell. https://www.eatingwell.com/recipe/274008/mediterranean-ravioli-with-artichokes-olives/

Hodges, C. A. (2019b, December). *Lemon-Roasted vegetable hummus bowls.* EatingWell. https://www.eatingwell.com/recipe/277634/lemon-roasted-vegetable-hummus-bowls/

Hodges, C. A. (2019c, December). *Sweet potato, kale & chicken salad with peanut dressing.* EatingWell. https://www.eatingwell.com/recipe/277650/sweet-potato-kale-chicken-salad-with-peanut-dressing/

Hoenselaar, R. (2012). Saturated fat and cardiovascular disease: The discrepancy between the scientific literature and dietary advice. *Nutrition,* 28, 118–123. https://doi.org/10.1016/j.nut.2011.08.017

I Breathe I'm Hungry. (2012, January 2). *Cream cheese pancakes - low carb & gluten free.* https://www.ibreatheimhungry.com/cream-cheese-pancakes/

I Breathe I'm Hungry. (2013a, August 28). *Easy cheesy cauliflower gratin recipe (low carb and gluten free).* https://www.ibreatheimhungry.com/cheesy-cauliflower-gratin-recipe-low-carb-and-gluten-free/

I Breathe I'm Hungry. (2013b, October 17). *Keto Latin American pot roast - low carb.* https://www.ibreatheimhungry.com/cuban-pot-roast-recipe-low-carb-gluten-free/

I Breathe I'm Hungry. (2013c, December 11). *Keto cheesy chili spaghetti squash casserole.* https://www.ibreatheimhungry.com/cheesy-chili-spaghetti-squash-casserole-low-carb-gluten-free/

I Breathe I'm Hungry. (2014, January 9). *Easy low carb egg salad and day one back on keto.* https://www.ibreatheimhungry.com/easy-low-carb-egg-salad-day-one-back-keto/

Iyer, S. (2016, April 6). *The pros and cons of going vegan.* SELF. https://www.self.com/story/vegan-diet-pros-cons

Jackson-Cannady, A. (2013, December 11). *The dukan diet.* WebMD. https://www.webmd.com/diet/a-z/dukan-diet

Johnson, J. (2019, January 18). *Our guide to the Mediterranean diet.* Www.medicalnewstoday.com. https://www.medicalnewstoday.com/articles/324221

Jones, T. (2017, February 14). *The raw food diet: A beginner's guide and review.* Healthline. https://www.healthline.com/nutrition/raw-food-diet

Killeen, B. (2017, August). *Lemon-Herb salmon with caponata & farro.* EatingWell. https://www.eatingwell.com/recipe/258522/lemon-herb-salmon-with-caponata-farro/

Killeen, B. (2019, March). *Beefless vegan tacos.* EatingWell. https://www.eatingwell.com/recipe/272203/beefless-vegan-tacos/

Killeen, B. (2021, January 4). *How to start juicing: 7-Day juice plan to add more fruits and vegetables to your diet.* EatingWell. https://www.eatingwell.com/article/278357/how-to-start-juicing-7-day-juice-plan-to-add-more-fruits-and-vegetables-to-your-diet/

Konstantinovsky, M. (2014, February 3). *7 days of juice recipes.* Www.onemedical.com. https://www.onemedical.com/blog/eat-well/7-juice-recipes

Krampf, M. (2017, September 6). *Bulletproof coffee recipe with MCT oil (the best keto butter coffee!).* Wholesome Yum. https://www.wholesomeyum.com/recipes/keto-butter-coffee-recipe-with-mct-oil/

Kylie. (2020, June 22). *Vegetarian Mediterranean lasagna.* Midwest Foodie. https://midwestfoodieblog.com/mediterranean-lasagna/#tasty-recipes-22793-jump-target

Lachtrupp, E. (2020a, February 24). *30-Day Mediterranean diet meal plan: 1,200 calories.* EatingWell.

https://www.eatingwell.com/article/291946/30-day-
mediterranean-diet-meal-plan-1200-calories/

Lachtrupp, E. (2020b, September 14). *Low cholesterol diet plan for beginners.*
EatingWell.
https://www.eatingwell.com/article/7836633/high-
cholesterol-diet-plan-for-beginners/

Lawler, M. (2019, April 22). *What is the raw vegan diet? Benefits, risks, meal
plan, and food list.* EverydayHealth.com.
https://www.everydayhealth.com/diet-nutrition/diet/raw-
vegan-diet-benefits-risks-meal-plan-food-list/

Leech, J. (2017, June 17). *The military diet: A beginner's guide (with a meal
plan).* Healthline. https://www.healthline.com/nutrition/the-
military-diet-101

Link, R. (2018, October 17). *The vegetarian diet: A beginner's guide and meal
plan.* Healthline;
https://www.healthline.com/nutrition/vegetarian-diet-plan

Link, R. (2019a, April 4). *A complete vegan meal plan and sample menu.*
Healthline. https://www.healthline.com/nutrition/vegan-meal-
plan

Link, R. (2019b, September 3). *Vegetarian keto diet plan: Benefits, risks, food
lists, and more.* Healthline.
https://www.healthline.com/nutrition/vegetarian-keto-diet-
plan

López-Alt, J. K. (2020, April 18). *Crispy vegan smoked-mushroom "bacon"
recipe.* Seriouseats.com.
https://www.seriouseats.com/recipes/2014/02/crispy-
smoked-mushroom-bacon-bits-vegan-recipe.html

Madigan, M., & Karhu, E. (2018). The role of plant-based nutrition in
cancer prevention. *Journal of Unexplored Medical Data*, 3, 9.
https://doi.org/10.20517/2572-8180.2018.05

Malcoun, C. (2019, March). *Slow-Cooker Mediterranean chicken & chickpea soup*. EatingWell. https://www.eatingwell.com/recipe/270484/slow-cooker-mediterranean-chicken-chickpea-soup/

Marcin, A. (2019, March 8). *The beginner's guide to becoming a vegetarian*. Healthline. https://www.healthline.com/health/becoming-vegetarian

Marshall, B. (2018, September 10). *The pros and cons of a keto diet*. Crisp Regional Hospital. https://crispregional.org/the-pros-and-cons-of-a-keto-diet/

Mayo Clinic Staff. (2016a). *6 proven strategies for weight-loss success*. Mayo Clinic. https://www.mayoclinic.org/healthy-lifestyle/weight-loss/in-depth/weight-loss/art-20047752

Mayo Clinic Staff. (2016b). *DASH diet: Healthy eating to lower your blood pressure*. Mayo Clinic. https://www.mayoclinic.org/healthy-lifestyle/nutrition-and-healthy-eating/in-depth/dash-diet/art-20048456

Mayo Clinic Staff. (2018). *Sample menus for the DASH diet*. Mayo Clinic. https://www.mayoclinic.org/healthy-lifestyle/nutrition-and-healthy-eating/in-depth/dash-diet/art-20047110

Mayo Clinic Staff. (2019). *Mediterranean diet: A heart-healthy eating plan*. Mayo Clinic https://www.mayoclinic.org/healthy-lifestyle/nutrition-and-healthy-eating/in-depth/mediterranean-diet/art-20047801

Mayo Clinic Staff. (n.d.). *HDL cholesterol: How to boost your "good" cholesterol*. Mayo Clinic; Retrieved March 25, 2021, from https://www.mayoclinic.org/diseases-conditions/high-blood-cholesterol/in-depth/hdl-cholesterol/art-20046388

McCallum, K. (2020, January 6). *Are juice cleanses actually good for you?* Www.houstonmethodist.org.

https://www.houstonmethodist.org/blog/articles/2020/jan/ar
e-juices-cleanses-actually-good-for-you/

McPhillips, K. (2020, August 12). *The 8 types of vegetarians all get down with plant-based eating in different ways.* Well+Good. https://www.wellandgood.com/types-of-vegetarians/

Meal Plans. (2004, May). *The CrossFit Journal, Issue 21*: 1–10. https://www.google.com/url?sa=t&rct=j&q=&esrc=s&source =web&cd=&cad=rja&uact=8&ved=2ahUKEwj28Kiuhd3vAh WNYcAKHQmSCdEQFjAbegQINRAD&url=https%3A%2F %2Flibrary.crossfit.com%2Ffree%2Fpdf%2Fcfjissue21_May04 .pdf&usg=AOvVaw0_6C-l2XeIu1bDWv9Wy_GB

Meyer, H. (2018, February). *Greek turkey burgers with spinach, feta & tzatziki.* EatingWell. https://www.eatingwell.com/recipe/262569/greek-turkey-burgers-with-spinach-feta-tzatziki/

Military Diet. (n.d.). *Military diet | 3 day diet.* Retrieved March 29, 2021, from https://themilitarydiet.com/

Miller, K. (n.d.). *Raw massaged kale salad with fresh figs and oranges [vegan].* One Green Planet. Retrieved April 3, 2021, from https://www.onegreenplanet.org/vegan-recipe/raw-massaged-kale-salad-with-fresh-figs-and-oranges/

Morris, J. (2013, July 11). *A green smoothie recipe.* The Chalkboard. https://thechalkboardmag.com/julie-morris-mint-chip-superfood-green-smoothie-recipe

My Dukan Diet. (2010a, September 13). *Dukan mayonnaise.* https://mydukandiet.com/recipes/dukan-mayonnaise.html

My Dukan Diet. (2010b, September 13). *Vietnamese beef.* https://mydukandiet.com/recipes/vietnamese-beef.html

My Dukan Diet. (n.d.-a). *Cinnamon pancakes.* Retrieved April 3, 2021, from https://mydukandiet.com/recipes/cinnamon-pancakes.html

My Dukan Diet. (n.d.-b). *Example menu for the dukan diet attack phase.* Retrieved April 2, 2021, from https://mydukandiet.com/dieting/example-menu-for-the-dukan-diet-attack-phase.html

My Dukan Diet. (n.d.-c). *Garlic tiger prawns.* Retrieved April 3, 2021, from https://mydukandiet.com/recipes/garlic-tiger-prawns.html

My Dukan Diet. (n.d.-d). *Muesli ice-cream.* Retrieved April 3, 2021, from https://mydukandiet.com/recipes/muesli-ice-cream.html

My Dukan Diet. (n.d.-e). *Oat bran cookies.* Retrieved April 3, 2021, from https://mydukandiet.com/recipes/oat-bran-cookies.html

My Dukan Diet. (n.d.-f). *Pink cheesecake cupcakes.* Retrieved April 3, 2021, from https://mydukandiet.com/recipes/pink-cheesecake-cupcakes.html

My Gut Health Today. (2018, July 25). *Pros and cons of the DASH diet.* https://www.myguthealthtoday.com/dash-diet-pros-cons/

My Plate. (n.d.). *My Plate low-fat meal search.* Www.myplate.gov. Retrieved April 1, 2021, from https://www.myplate.gov/search?keyword=low%20fat&page=0

Nall, R. (2018, September 21). *Juice cleanse: Benefits, risks, and effects.* Www.medicalnewstoday.com. https://www.medicalnewstoday.com/articles/323136

Nall, R. (2019, July 25). *Low fat foods: List, benefits, and meal plan.* Www.medicalnewstoday.com. https://www.medicalnewstoday.com/articles/325860

Nettleton, J. A., Brouwer, I. A., Geleijnse, J. M., & Hornstra, G. (2017). Saturated Fat Consumption and Risk of Coronary Heart Disease and Ischemic Stroke: A Science Update. *Annals of Nutrition & Metabolism, 70*, 26–33. https://doi.org/10.1159/000455681

Nicole. (2015, May 14). *One-Day At-Home Green Juice Reset (+Grocery List).* Pumps & Iron. https://pumpsandiron.com/2015/05/14/one-day-at-home-green-juice-reset-grocery-list/

Northwestern Medicine Staff. (2019, January 2). *Pros and cons of the ketogenic diet.* Northwestern Medicine. https://www.nm.org/healthbeat/healthy-tips/nutrition/pros-and-cons-of-ketogenic-diet

O'Brien, D. (2017, February). *Vegan pancakes.* EatingWell. https://www.eatingwell.com/recipe/257348/vegan-pancakes/

Oberg, E. (2020, February 9). *DASH diet eating plan: Foods to avoid & foods to eat.* MedicineNet. https://www.medicinenet.com/the_dash_diet/article.htm

Olive Tomato. (2018, July 23). *The complete Mediterranean diet food and shopping list.* https://www.olivetomato.com/the-complete-mediterranean-diet-food-shopping-list/

One Green Planet. (n.d.). *Plant-Based weekly meal plan by diet: Raw vegan menu.* Retrieved April 2, 2021, from https://www.onegreenplanet.org/vegan-food/weekly-meal-plan-the-raw-vegan-menu/

Pasquale, N. (2013, March 12). *Juice cleanse guide for successful cleansing.* Urban Remedy. https://urbanremedy.com/how-to-do-a-juice-cleanse/

Pearson, K. (2017, May 16). *Is pink Himalayan salt better than regular salt?* Healthline. https://www.healthline.com/nutrition/pink-himalayan-salt

Petre, A. (2016, November 1). *The vegan diet — A complete guide for beginners.* Healthline. https://www.healthline.com/nutrition/vegan-diet-guide

Petre, A. (2018, December 3). *How to follow a raw vegan diet: Benefits and risks.* Healthline. https://www.healthline.com/nutrition/raw-vegan-diet

Petre, A. (2020, February 28). *Are figs vegan?* Healthline. https://www.healthline.com/nutrition/are-figs-vegan

Petrova, N. (n.d.). *Raw blackberry breakfast chocolate cake [vegan].* One Green Planet. Retrieved April 3, 2021, from https://www.onegreenplanet.org/vegan-recipe/raw-blackberry-breakfast-chocolate-cake/

Plenty Vegan. (2016, November 27). *Vegan grocery list for beginners.* https://plentyvegan.com/vegan-grocery-list-for-beginners/

Pritikin. (2016). *Diet plan to lower cholesterol and lose weight.* Pritikin.com. https://www.pritikin.com/best-meal-plan-for-lower-cholesterol

Project Juice. (n.d.). *How to do a juice cleanse.* Projectjuice.com. Retrieved March 28, 2021, from https://www.projectjuice.com/how-to-cleanse

Raman, R. (2017, April 4). *The zone diet: A complete overview.* Healthline. https://www.healthline.com/nutrition/zone-diet

Reyzelman, A. (2017, August 15). *Advantages and disadvantages of a low-fat diet.* EatWellCo. http://www.eatwellco.com/2017/08/advantages-and-disadvantages-of-a-low-fat-diet/

Robertson, S. (2017, August 16). *New Atkins diet: Pros and cons.* News-Medical.net. https://www.news-medical.net/health/New-Atkins-Diet-Pros-and-Cons.aspx

Robinson, K. M. (2013, December 11). *Raw foods diet*. WebMD. https://www.webmd.com/diet/a-z/raw-foods-diet

Ruled Me. (2013, October 9). *Keto recipe: Fluffy buttermilk pancakes*. https://www.ruled.me/fluffy-buttermilk-pancakes/

Ruled Me. (2014, October 27). *Pumpkin spiced french toast*. https://www.ruled.me/pumpkin-spiced-french-toast/

Ruled Me. (2016, December 22). *Keto cookies and crème ice cream*. https://www.ruled.me/keto-cookies-creme-ice-cream/

Ruled Me. (2017a, February 9). *Keto vanilla bean cupcakes*. https://www.ruled.me/keto-vanilla-bean-cupcakes/

Ruled Me. (2017b, June 15). *Zucchini ribbons & avocado walnut pesto*. https://www.ruled.me/zucchini-ribbons-with-avocado-walnut-pesto/

Ruled Me. (2017c, August 8). *Low carb coconut chip cookies*. https://www.ruled.me/low-carb-coconut-chip-cookies/

Ruled Me. (2017d, September 14). *Garlic and herb monkey "bread."* https://www.ruled.me/garlic-herb-monkey-bread/

Ruled Me. (2017e, October 3). *Charred veggie and fried goat cheese salad*. https://www.ruled.me/charred-veggie-fried-goat-cheese-salad/

Ruled Me. (2017f, October 10). *Tropical chocolate mousse bites*. https://www.ruled.me/tropical-chocolate-mousse-bites/

Sarah. (2018, October 26). *Vegan keto chocolate fat bombs (sugar free + low carb)*. Vegan Chickpea. https://veganchickpea.com/vegan-keto-chocolate-fat-bombs-sugar-free-low-carb/

Satterthwaite, L. (2018, December 11). *The pros and cons of the keto diet*. Promedicahealthconnect.org.

https://promedicahealthconnect.org/wellness/the-pros-and-cons-of-the-keto-diet/

Science Daily. (2019, September 4). *Long-term benefits of a low-fat diet.* https://www.sciencedaily.com/releases/2019/09/1909040903 02.htm

Scott, J. R. (2020, November 2). *Atkins diet pros and cons.* Verywell Fit. https://www.verywellfit.com/pros-and-cons-of-the-atkins-diet-3496221

Seaver, V. (2017a, November). *Peanut butter-banana cinnamon toast.* EatingWell. https://www.eatingwell.com/recipe/261628/peanut-butter-banana-cinnamon-toast/

Seaver, V. (2017b, November). *Roasted veggie & quinoa salad.* EatingWell. https://www.eatingwell.com/recipe/261290/roasted-veggie-quinoa-salad/

Seaver, V. (2017c, November). *White bean & avocado toast.* EatingWell. https://www.eatingwell.com/recipe/261611/white-bean-avocado-toast/

Seaver, V. (2019, December 11). *7-Day vegan meal plan: 1,200 calories.* EatingWell. https://www.eatingwell.com/article/290194/7-day-vegan-meal-plan-1200-calories/

Seaver, V. (2020a, January 10). *7-Day DASH diet menu.* EatingWell. https://www.eatingwell.com/article/289964/7-day-dash-diet-menu/

Seaver, V. (2020b, February 17). *7-Day vegetarian meal plan: 1,500 calories.* EatingWell. https://www.eatingwell.com/article/289024/7-day-vegetarian-meal-plan-1500-calories/

Seaver, V. (2020c, February 18). *7-Day diet meal plan to lose weight: 1,500 calories.* EatingWell.

https://www.eatingwell.com/article/287714/7-day-diet-meal-plan-to-lose-weight-1500-calories/

Sevigny, M. (2014, January 10). *Week one keto/low carb 7 day meal plan & progress.* I Breathe I'm Hungry. https://www.ibreatheimhungry.com/week-one-ketolow-carb-7-day-meal-plan-progress/

Slajerova, M. (2019, September 29). *2 week vegetarian keto diet plan.* KetoDiet. https://ketodietapp.com/Blog/lchf/2-week-vegetarian-keto-diet-plan

Slajerova, M. (2020a, March 22). *Low-Carb egg stuffed avocado.* KetoDiet. https://ketodietapp.com/Blog/lchf/egg-stuffed-avocado

Slajerova, M. (2020b, March 22). *Quick frittata with tomatoes and cheese.* KetoDiet. https://ketodietapp.com/Blog/lchf/quick-frittata-with-tomatoes-and-cheese

Slajerova, M. (2020c, March 22). *Vegetarian keto lasagna.* KetoDiet. https://ketodietapp.com/Blog/lchf/vegetarian-keto-lasagna

Slajerova, M. (2020d, September 7). *Easy avocado & egg salad.* KetoDiet. https://ketodietapp.com/Blog/lchf/easy-avocado-and-egg-salad

Slajerova, M. (2020e, October 7). *Chocolate keto smoothie.* KetoDiet. https://ketodietapp.com/Blog/lchf/Chocolate-Keto-Smoothie

Slajerova, M. (2020f, October 9). *Classic tricolore salad.* KetoDiet. https://ketodietapp.com/Blog/lchf/classic-tricolore-salad

Slajerova, M. (2021, March 11). *Low-Carb pesto egg muffins.* KetoDiet. https://ketodietapp.com/Blog/lchf/pesto-egg-muffins

Smith, A. N. (2015, February 2). *Raw vegan chocolate chip cookies.* https://amandanicolesmith.com/raw-vegan-chocolate-chip-cookies/

Sorai, C., & Laderman, D. (n.d.). *Raw food for dummies cheat sheet.* Dummies. Retrieved March 27, 2021, from https://www.dummies.com/health/nutrition/raw-food-for-dummies-cheat-sheet/

Spaeder, K. (2019, October 23). *Atkins diet & phase 1 meal plans.* LIVESTRONG.COM. https://www.livestrong.com/article/388086-atkins-diet-phase-1-meal-plans/

Spritzler, F. (2018, December 12). *The dukan diet review: Does it work for weight loss?* Healthline. https://www.healthline.com/nutrition/dukan-diet-101

Spritzler, F. (2021, March 7). *Keto and low-carb dairy: The best and the worst.* Diet Doctor. https://www.dietdoctor.com/low-carb/keto/dairy

Strong, R. (2020, December 24). *Cut back on meat for a week with this 7-day vegetarian meal plan recommended by a registered dietitian.* Insider. https://www.insider.com/vegetarian-meal-plan

Sundblad, D. (n.d.). *How long should you stay on the Atkins diet?* LoveToKnow. Retrieved March 25, 2021, from https://diet.lovetoknow.com/wiki/How_Long_Should_You_Stay_on_the_Atkins_Diet

Taste of Home. (n.d.-a). *Arborio rice and white bean soup.* Retrieved April 3, 2021, from https://www.tasteofhome.com/recipes/arborio-rice-and-white-bean-soup/

Taste of Home. (n.d.-b). *Broccoli & chive stuffed mini peppers.* Retrieved April 3, 2021, from https://www.tasteofhome.com/recipes/broccoli-chive-stuffed-mini-peppers/

Taste of Home. (n.d.-c). *Family-Favorite oatmeal waffles.* Retrieved April 3, 2021, from https://www.tasteofhome.com/recipes/family-favorite-oatmeal-waffles/

Taste of Home. (n.d.-d). *Garden-Fresh grilled veggie pizza*. Retrieved April 3, 2021, from https://www.tasteofhome.com/recipes/garden-fresh-grilled-veggie-pizza/

Taste of Home. (n.d.-e). *Mediterranean bulgur bowl*. Retrieved April 3, 2021, from https://www.tasteofhome.com/recipes/mediterranean-bulgur-bowl/

Taste of Home. (n.d.-f). *Overnight baked eggs bruschetta*. Retrieved April 3, 2021, from https://www.tasteofhome.com/recipes/overnight-baked-eggs-bruschetta/

Taste of Home. (n.d.-g). *Pepper ricotta primavera*. Retrieved April 3, 2021, from https://www.tasteofhome.com/recipes/pepper-ricotta-primavera/

Taste of Home. (n.d.-h). *Portobello mushrooms florentine*. Retrieved April 3, 2021, from https://www.tasteofhome.com/recipes/portobello-mushrooms-florentine/

Taste of Home. (n.d.-i). *Powerhouse protein parfaits*. Retrieved April 3, 2021, from https://www.tasteofhome.com/recipes/powerhouse-protein-parfaits/

Taste of Home. (n.d.-j). *Roasted beetroot and garlic hummus*. Retrieved April 3, 2021, from https://www.tasteofhome.com/recipes/roasted-beetroot-and-garlic-hummus/

Taste of Home. (n.d.-k). *Roasted sweet potato & chickpea pitas*. Retrieved April 3, 2021, from https://www.tasteofhome.com/recipes/roasted-sweet-potato-chickpea-pitas/

The Best Dash Diet Recipes. (2019, February 26). *Herbs and spices*. https://bestdashdietrecipes.wordpress.com/about/healthy-snacks/herbs-and-spices/

The Chalkboard. (2013a, August 29). *Smoothie solutions: Belly blaster smoothie recipe.* https://thechalkboardmag.com/smoothie-solutions-the-berry-belly-blaster

The Chalkboard. (2013b, October 15). *Rustic autumn roasted apples with roots and greens.* https://thechalkboardmag.com/organic-garden-tour-an-eco-resort-on-the-mendocino-coast#sl=1

The Chalkboard. (2013c, October 24). *Persimmon salad recipe.* https://thechalkboardmag.com/first-of-the-season-raw-pistachio-persimmon-salad

The Chalkboard. (2014, January 2). *Getting started: Pre-Cleanse food menu.* https://thechalkboardmag.com/getting-started-pre-cleanse-food-menu

The Iron You. (2016, June 24). *Zoodles with creamy garlic cashew sauce.* https://www.theironyou.com/2016/06/zoodles-with-creamy-garlic-cashew-sauce.html

The Portland Clinic. (2020, January 15). *The keto diet: Pros, cons and tips.* https://www.theportlandclinic.com/the-keto-diet-pros-cons-and-tips/

The Simple Veganista. (2012, July 19). *Raw pad thai (healthy + easy recipe).* https://simple-veganista.com/raw-pad-thai/

The Simple Veganista. (2020, June 1). *Walnut meat (healthy + easy).* https://simple-veganista.com/walnut-meat/#tasty-recipes-38662-jump-target

U.S. Department of Agriculture and U.S. Department of Health and Human Services. (2020). *Dietary Guidelines for Americans, 2020-2025.* 9th Edition.

USDA My Plate. (n.d.-a). *Cauliflower shells with cheese.* Www.myplate.gov. Retrieved April 3, 2021, from https://www.myplate.gov/recipes/supplemental-nutrition-assistance-program-snap/cauliflower-shells-cheese

USDA My Plate. (n.d.-b). *Cream of broccoli soup*. Www.myplate.gov. Retrieved April 3, 2021, from https://www.myplate.gov/recipes/supplemental-nutrition-assistance-program-snap/cream-broccoli-soup-ii

USDA My Plate. (n.d.-c). *Grape and cashew salad sandwich*. Www.myplate.gov. Retrieved April 3, 2021, from https://www.myplate.gov/recipes/myplate-cnpp/grape-and-cashew-salad-sandwich

USDA My Plate. (n.d.-d). *Yogurt berry parfait*. Www.myplate.gov. Retrieved April 3, 2021, from https://www.myplate.gov/recipes/supplemental-nutrition-assistance-program-snap/yogurt-berry-parfait

Valente, L. (2014, October). *Pineapple green smoothie*. EatingWell. https://www.eatingwell.com/recipe/251038/pineapple-green-smoothie/

Vegetarian Times Editors. (2007, June 16). *Why go veg?* Vegetarian Times. https://www.vegetariantimes.com/health-nutrition/why-go-veg-learn-about-becoming-a-vegetarian/

Velasquez, M. (2005, March). *Chocolate & nut butter bites*. EatingWell. https://www.eatingwell.com/recipe/248913/chocolate-nut-butter-bites/

Veronika's Kitchen. (2020, November 12). *No bake energy bites*. https://veronikaskitchen.com/no-bake-energy-bites-dates-nuts/

Vespa, J. (2019, May). *Mushroom-Quinoa veggie burgers with special sauce*. EatingWell. https://www.eatingwell.com/recipe/273896/mushroom-quinoa-veggie-burgers-with-special-sauce/

Von Euw, E. (n.d.-a). *Berry chia smoothie with cacao drizzle [vegan]*. One Green Planet. Retrieved April 3, 2021, from https://www.onegreenplanet.org/vegan-recipe/breakfast-berry-smoothie-with-cacao-drizzle-and-chia-pudding/

Von Euw, E. (n.d.-b). *Creamy and raw butternut squash soup with marinated mushrooms*. One Green Planet. Retrieved April 3, 2021, from https://www.onegreenplanet.org/vegan-recipe/creamy-raw-butternut-squash-soup-with-marinated-mushrooms/

Von Euw, E. (n.d.-c). *Raw enchiladas* [vegan]. One Green Planet. Retrieved April 3, 2021, from https://www.onegreenplanet.org/vegan-recipe/enchiladas-with-chunky-salsa-cheesy-sauce-and-spicy-nut-meat/

Von Euw, E. (n.d.-d). *Raw pizza [vegan]*. One Green Planet. Retrieved April 3, 2021, from https://www.onegreenplanet.org/vegan-recipe/ultimate-raw-vegan-pizza-low-fat-oil-free-salt-free/

Waygood, J. (2019, August 22). *DASH diet shopping list for phase 1 and beyond*. Listonic. https://listonic.com/dash-diet-shopping-list/

WebMD. (2020, March 16). *Foods that may help with muscle cramps*. https://www.webmd.com/pain-management/ss/slideshow-muscle-cramps-foods

Webster, K. (2017a, August). *Green salad with edamame & beets*. EatingWell. https://www.eatingwell.com/recipe/259814/green-salad-with-edamame-beets/

Webster, K. (2017b, August). *Veggie & hummus sandwich*. EatingWell. https://www.eatingwell.com/recipe/259817/veggie-hummus-sandwich/

Webster, K. (2017c, August). *White bean & veggie salad*. EatingWell. https://www.eatingwell.com/recipe/259819/white-bean-veggie-salad/

Webster, K. (2017d, August). *Whole-Wheat veggie wrap*. EatingWell. https://www.eatingwell.com/recipe/259820/whole wheat-veggie-wrap/

Webster, K. (2017e, October). *Black bean-quinoa buddha bowl*. EatingWell. https://www.eatingwell.com/recipe/260726/black-bean-quinoa-buddha-bowl/

Webster, K. (2017f, October). *Stuffed sweet potato with hummus dressing*. EatingWell. https://www.eatingwell.com/recipe/260717/stuffed-sweet-potato-with-hummus-dressing/

West, H. (2018, October 17). *The complete beginner's guide to the DASH diet*. Healthline. https://www.healthline.com/nutrition/dash-diet

WOD Fever. (n.d.). *The ultimate zone diet food list*. Retrieved March 26, 2021, from https://wodfever.com/blogs/new-posts/the-ultimate-zone-diet-food-list

Wong, C. (2021, January 16). *What is a juice cleanse?* Verywell Fit. https://www.verywellfit.com/juice-cleanse-89120

Yetman, D. (2020, December 4). *Fat deficiency: 5 signs of too little fat in your diet*. Healthline. https://www.healthline.com/health/fat-deficiency

York, J. (n.d.). *Raw triple berry cheesecake [vegan]*. One Green Planet. Retrieved April 3, 2021, from https://www.onegreenplanet.org/vegan-recipe/triple-berry-cheesecake/

Young, L. (2012, March 28). *Juice cleanse shopping list + recipes + schedule*. Lacy Young. https://www.lacyyoung.com/blog/juice/juice-cleanse/juice-cleanse-shopping-list-recipes-schedule

Image References

Castrejon, E. (2017, November 26). *Mediterranean cuisine is always bursting with color and flavor. It is no wonder people love it.* Unsplash. https://unsplash.com/photos/1SPu0KT-Ejg

Chung, Z. (2020, October 05). *Why not take a pleasant trip to a farm to pick the fruit for your dishes yourself? Exercise and a snack all rolled into one!* Pexels. https://www.pexels.com/photo/mother-and-daughter-walking-together-near-apple-trees-5528997/

Fador, D. (2013, October 02). *Walking is not only rewarding when it comes to the view it also works off those excess calories so that you can enjoy your meals guilt-free.* Pixabay. https://pixabay.com/photos/dog-mountain-mombarone-clouds-190056/

Free-Photos. (2015, November 9). *Visit a butcher to get the best deals on all the meat you will need for this diet.* Pixabay. https://pixabay.com/photos/meat-butcher-display-showcase-1030729/

Hamra, J. (2018, August 7). *A standard keto breakfast.* Pexels. https://www.pexels.com/photo/egg-near-blueberries-1305063/

K15 Photos. (2019, February 24). *Whether you choose juice or blend these drinks are always bursting with color and flavor.* Unsplash. https://unsplash.com/photos/YgKmmIVAj8E

Lach, R. (2021, February 16) *Deliciously prepared meal.* Pexels. https://www.pexels.com/photo/bread-food-toast-party-6954466/

McCarty, D.T. (2020, June 14). *A diet isn't just about food. It is a lifestyle change. It is something anyone can do if they put their mind to it. The more support you have the easier it will be.* Unsplash. https://unsplash.com/photos/TUUEdIhwNFQ

MootikaLLC. (2017, May 26). *Missing pasta on the Atkins diet? Zucchini noodles make for an excellent substitute.* Pixabay. https://pixabay.com/photos/zucchini-noodle-noodles-zoodle-2340977/

Olsson, E. (2018, November 03). *Nutrient-packed vegetarian lunch.* Pexels. https://www.pexels.com/photo/fruit-salads-in-plate-1640774/

Oquendo, C. (2019, October 03). *Is the convenience of junk food worth the health cost?* Pexels. https://www.pexels.com/photo/top-view-photo-of-food-3023476/

Palacio, E. (2019, May 29). *A perfect vegan breakfast.* Pixabay. https://pixabay.com/photos/breakfast-fruit-food-healthy-4234047/

Pixabay. (2017, June 05). *If the juice diet is a little difficult then make use of healthy smoothies.* Pexels. https://www.pexels.com/photo/berries-blackberries-close-up-cocktail-434295/

Primeau, N. (2018a, October 25). *A bowl full of colorful, raw vegetables and fruits, ready to be enjoyed immediately.* Unsplash. https://unsplash.com/photos/-ftWfohtjNw

Primeau, N. (2018b, November 21). *Low sodium doesn't mean boring. A salad can gain flavor with the use of onions, chilis, and lemon juice.* Unsplash. https://unsplash.com/photos/KD3XqquHlcc

Raic, V. (2014, July 30). *The scale doesn't define who you! Eat healthy to discover who you are.* Pixabay. https://pixabay.com/photos/scale-diet-fat-health-tape-weight-403585/

Shevtsova, D. (2018, October 14). *Farmers' markets are bursting with color and a variety of fruits and vegetables you can use.* Pexels.

https://www.pexels.com/photo/variety-of-vegetables-on-display-1508666/

Wow_Pho. (2016, April 21). *A grilled chicken breast with a side salad and half a lemon for taste, a perfect low-fat meal.* Pixabay. https://pixabay.com/photos/grilled-chicken-quinoa-salad-1334632/

Yahya, D.P.A. (2020, July 4). *Sprouting your own lentils are as easy as planting and watering the seeds until they start to grow.* Unsplash. https://unsplash.com/photos/Dj3aCuVxAS4

Yousaf, U. (2020, August 25). *A mixture of different nuts give a healthy dose of fats and proteins to all who enjoy them.* Unsplash. https://unsplash.com/photos/bvQ2hgDzjFA